PRINCIPLES OF NLP

other titles in the series

PRINCIPLES OF
THE ALEXANDER TECHNIQUE
Jeremy Chance

PRINCIPLES OF
BACH FLOWER REMEDIES
Stefan Ball

PRINCIPLES OF
CHINESE HERBAL MEDICINE
John Hicks

PRINCIPLES OF
CHINESE MEDICINE
Angela Hicks

PRINCIPLES OF
THE ENNEAGRAM
Karen A. Webb

PRINCIPLES OF
HYPNOTHERAPY
Vera Peiffer

PRINCIPLES OF
KINESIOLOGY
Maggie La Tourelle with Anthea Courtenay

PRINCIPLES OF
REFLEXOLOGY
Nicola Hall

PRINCIPLES OF
REIKI
Kajsa Krishni Boräng

PRINCIPLES OF
TIBETAN MEDICINE
Dr. Tamdin Sither Bradley

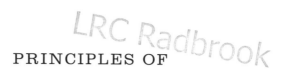

PRINCIPLES OF

NLP

What it is, how it works, and what it can do for you

Revised Edition

Joseph O'Connor and Ian McDermott

Foreword by Robert Dilts

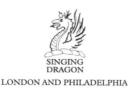

SINGING
DRAGON

LONDON AND PHILADELPHIA

This edition published in 2013
by Singing Dragon
an imprint of Jessica Kingsley Publishers
116 Pentonville Road
London N1 9JB, UK
and
400 Market Street, Suite 400
Philadelphia, PA 19106, USA

www.singingdragon.com

First published in 1996 by Thorsons, an imprint of HarperCollins

Library of Congress Cataloging in Publication Data
A CIP catalog record for this book is available from the Library of Congress

British Library Cataloguing in Publication Data
A CIP catalogue record for this book is available from the British Library

ISBN 978 1 84819 161 7
eISBN 978 0 85701 136 7

Printed and bound in Great Britain

To our parents

CONTENTS

Foreword

It has been many years now since I first became exposed to the ideas and methods that were to grow into the field of 'NLP'. In those early days, there were none of the quick, 'slick' techniques that are associated with NLP today. Rather, there was a deep excitement about a new way to approach learning, choice and change. This excitement was fuelled by a set of unique and powerful presuppositions about human thought and behaviour that have been the generating principles of all of the developments of NLP that have followed.

The underlying mission of NLP has always been to unveil something about the 'deeper structure' of being a human being and the process by which those invisible structures are transformed into the surface structures which determine how we interact with the world. The 'deep structure' of NLP is its presuppositions.

By taking the NLP presuppositions as their starting-point, Joseph and Ian have emphasized the most generative aspect of NLP, and hopefully will help shift the focus of NLP interventions from simply behaviour and capability-level change to show its relevance for dealing with higher-level issues involving beliefs, identity and spirituality.

It is comforting to see the return to these roots of NLP after so many years of emphasis on surface results. I hope you are able to learn something more of the deep richness of NLP through the surface structure of this book.

Robert Dilts

ACKNOWLEDGEMENTS

Our thanks to all our teachers, and we want to give credit and recognition to John Grinder and Richard Bandler, co-developers of NLP, and to Robert Dilts, for contributing so much to the field. Milton Erickson is credited with embodying many of the principles in this book, and so we thank him for articulating them in action.

Thanks to our editor at Singing Dragon, Emily McClave, for bringing this edition into being.

As authors, we work together as equals, bringing together our skills into this project as we do in many others. Therefore the order in which the names appear on the cover of this book has no significance.

We hope this book furthers the growth and development of NLP in a positive way. We have learned much from writing it.

Introduction

The principles of NLP. It is a delight for us to write about them. NLP is practical, it is about experience – your experience; what it is, not what it should be. It is about enriching your own world-view.

What is NLP? Its title gives one answer. 'Neuro' refers to the mind and how we organize our mental life. 'Linguistic' is about language, how we use it and how it affects us. 'Programming' is about our sequences of repetitive behaviour and how we act with purpose. So NLP is about connection, for our thoughts, speech and actions are what connects us to others, the world and to the spiritual dimension.

This is a practical book, explaining how NLP translates into your everyday life. Although well grounded in psychological theory and research, NLP is first and foremost about action. It gives you more choices in your mind and body, and so frees you to explore spirit.

The starting-point of NLP is curiosity and fascination about people. It is the study of the structure of subjective experience. How do we do what we do? How do we think? How do we learn? How do we get angry? And how do outstanding people in any field get their results? To answer these questions NLP explores how we think and feel and studies or 'models' excellence in every walk of life. The answers can then be taught to others. The goal is excellence for all.

NLP began in the early 1970s when Richard Bandler, a student of psychology at the University of California, Santa Cruz, began working with John Grinder, then

Assistant Professor of Linguistics. Together they modelled three people: Fritz Perls, the innovative psychologist and originator of Gestalt therapy; Virginia Satir, the prime force behind family therapy; and Milton Erickson, the world famous hypnotherapist, whose ideas are continued in Ericksonian hypnotherapy. They also drew on the insights and ideas of many others, particularly Gregory Bateson, the British writer and thinker on anthropology, cybernetics and communications theory. Their first models dealt with verbal and non-verbal communication skills. Consequently, NLP has given rise to a trail of techniques that can be used both personally and professionally. They are used internationally in fields such as sports, business, sales and education, and enable us not only to reach out and influence others, but also to reach in and unify the different parts of our selves.

You will find these skills, and more, in this book. We have attempted to give you the process that created the techniques, so you can take the ideas and make them your own in the way that suits you best. NLP is a generative psychology. It is also 'the psychology of excellence'. It has a vision of a world in which there is no shortage of excellence and where education is about helping *everyone* to be outstanding.

Our body and mind seem constant, but are changing all the time, like a river – ceaseless activity, moment by moment change, yet overall something at a deep level is the same. Thoughts and physiology are intimately connected: what and how we think affect our physiology, and our physical health and well-being affect our thoughts.

Our mind, body and spirit meet in our beliefs. What we believe deeply affects what we think and how we act. NLP sees beliefs not in terms of true or false, but in terms of useful or not useful. What are the consequences of your beliefs? What actions flow from them? As we cannot know everything about the world, in many areas our beliefs are simply our best guess at the moment. We have a special invitation for you: we invite you to look at your beliefs and see how they serve you.

Sometimes what we do and what we believe do not match. This reminds us of a story. Many years ago, the Great Zumbrati had just completed a tightrope walk over the Niagara Falls. The conditions were bad, it was a blustery day and he was very glad when he stepped safely onto the other side to meet his public, an admiring crowd of well-wishers. One man was waiting holding a wheelbarrow.

'That was wonderful!' said the man. 'You are a master!'

The Great Zumbrati thanked him and said that the weather had made the crossing very difficult.

'Nonsense,' said the man. 'I bet you could walk back across pushing this wheelbarrow.'

Zumbrati demurred. 'I don't think so,' he said. 'Conditions are too bad.'

The man, however, would not give up and kept urging him to do it. Zumbrati became exasperated.

'You really believe I could, don't you?' he asked the man.

'Yes.'

'Are you sure?'

'Yes.'

'OK. Get in the wheelbarrow.'

This book is arranged around the basic operating principles, or *presuppositions*, of NLP. They are called presuppositions because you presuppose them, that is, you act *as if* they were true and notice the results you get. They are actually working hypotheses that may or may not be literally true. NLP does not claim they are true. The question to ask is not 'Are they true?' but 'Are they useful?'

We have aimed here to give you the core of NLP, the concepts, the structure and the practical uses. We have also included examples from our own experience. Faced with an Aladdin's cave of possibilities, we have explored the main treasure trove and a few fascinating passageways. We hope you uncover some treasures here. For a more comprehensive map of Aladdin's cave, look in the bibliography section at the end of the book for suggestions on books to explore.

And now: 'Open Sesame…'

1

The Four Pillars of Wisdom

There are four main principles in NLP and we will be returning to them from different angles throughout this book. The first and foremost is relationship, specifically that quality relationship of mutual trust and responsiveness known as *rapport*. It can be applied both to your relationship with yourself and your relationship with others.

We begin with the rapport you have with yourself. You have probably felt torn between two courses of action at some time in your life. Have you ever heard yourself say things like, 'Part of me wants to do this, but something stops me'? The greater the degree of *physical* rapport you have with yourself, the greater your health and well-being, for the different parts of your body are working well with each other. The greater your *mental* rapport with yourself, the more you feel at peace with yourself, for the different parts of your mind are united. Rapport at the *spiritual* level can manifest as a sense of belonging to a larger whole, beyond individual identity, and knowing our place in creation.

There are many who have all the external trappings of success, yet are unhappy within themselves. You may have noticed that such people make others uneasy too. We seem to arrange the world in a way that reflects our internal state. So internal conflicts create external ones and the quality of the rapport we have with ourselves is often a mirror of what we achieve with others.

Whatever you do and whatever you want, being successful will involve relating to and influencing others. So the first pillar of NLP is to establish rapport with yourself and then others.

The second pillar is to know what you want. Without knowing what you want, you cannot even define what success is. In NLP this is known as setting your *goal* or *outcome*. It is a whole way of thinking. You consistently ask yourself, 'What do I want?' and others, 'What do you want?' This is very different from going in with a question like 'What's the problem?' Many people start by asking this question, then apportion blame and perhaps fix the situation, but never get what they really want or help others get what they really want either.

The third pillar is known as *sensory acuity*. This means using your senses: looking at, listening to and feeling what is actually happening to you. Only then will you know whether you are on course for your goal. You can use this feedback to adjust what you are doing if necessary. In this culture it is thought normal *not* to notice this kind of information. But children notice. We can regain the curiosity and acuity we had as children.

The last pillar is behavioural flexibility. Have many choices of action. The more choices you have, the more chance of success. Keep changing what you do until you get what you want. This sounds simple, even obvious, yet how many times do we do just the opposite? A government will often continue to pursue a policy even though it is clearly not having the desired effect. It also happens in relationships – have there been times when you and your partner were arguing and you could just see that you were getting into a hole, yet somehow you just kept digging?

Logical levels

We build relationships on different levels. The American researcher and NLP trainer Robert Dilts uses a series of what he calls *neurological levels* that have been widely adopted in NLP thinking. They are very useful for thinking about building rapport and personal change. The six levels are explained below and illustrated in Figure 1.1.

1. *Environment (the where and when)*. The environment is the place we are in and the people we are with. You have probably heard people say that they were in the 'right place at the right time'. They are attributing their success to their environment. At this level, shared circumstances build rapport. For example, if you were to go to an evening class about Chinese Art, you would expect to meet others with a similar interest. You would have a point of contact with each other and a basic degree of rapport.

2. *Behaviour (the what)*. This is the level of our specific, conscious actions: what we do. In NLP behaviour includes thoughts as well as actions. What we do is not random; our behaviour is designed to achieve a purpose, although this may not always be clear, even to us. We may want to change our behaviour, smoking or constantly losing our temper, for example. But sometimes unwanted behaviour may be difficult to change because it is closely connected with other neurological levels.

3. *Capability (the how)*. This is the level of skill: behaviour that we have practised so often it has become consistent, automatic and often habitual. This includes thinking strategies and physical skills. We all have many basic intrinsic skills, such as walking and talking, and also

consciously learnt skills, such as mathematics, sport or playing a musical instrument. When someone describes their success as a 'one-off' or a 'fluke', they are ascribing it to the level of behaviour only, they do not think it is repeatable consistently, and it is not yet a capability.

4. *Beliefs and values (the why).* This is the level of what we believe is true and what is important to us. Beliefs and values direct our lives to a considerable extent, acting both as permissions and prohibitions. Are there some skills you would like to develop, but think you can't? As long as you believe you can't, you won't. Is there a skill you need to learn but don't consider important? If you don't value it, you will never be motivated enough to acquire it. We are also capable of holding conflicting beliefs and values, resulting in actions that contradict each other over time.

5. *Identity (the who).* Have you heard someone say something like 'I am just not that kind of person'? That is an identity statement. Identity is your sense of yourself, your core beliefs and values that define who you are and your mission in life. Your identity is very resilient, although you can build, develop and change it.

6. *Spirituality.* This is your connection to others and to that which is more than your identity, however you choose to think of it. Rapport at this level is described in spiritual literature as being one with humankind, the universe or God.

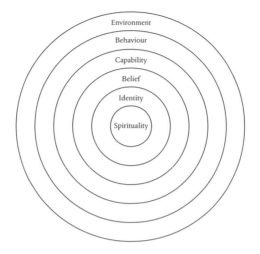

Figure 1.1 Logical levels

When NLP was developed in the early 1970s, there was a gap in psychological thinking. The Behaviourist psychology of the time was about action and reaction, stimulus-response, and the interaction between environment and behaviour. There were also many value-based psychological systems, stressing beliefs, relationships and self-actualization. What was conspicuously missing was how to – the capability level. NLP stepped into this gap by providing step-by-step procedures to make excellence easily learnable.

Behaviour to capability

How does behaviour become a skill? One answer is the reply given to the man carrying a violin who asked the way to Carnegie Hall: 'Practise.'

Learning a skill goes through four stages. Think of some intentional skill that you have acquired in the course of your life – driving, riding a bicycle or reading – and see how it fits into this scheme. You start from *unconscious incompetence.* In this state, not only can you not do it, you have never tried. You don't even know that you don't know.

Then you start to do it. At first, although it is part of your behaviour, you are not very skilled. This is the stage of *conscious incompetence.* You know enough to know you are not very good and it takes a lot of your conscious attention. This stage is uncomfortable, but it is also when you are learning the most.

Next you reach the stage of *conscious competence.* You can do it, you have reached the capability level, but it still takes a lot of your attention.

Lastly, if you persevere, you reach the stage of *unconscious competence*, when you do it easily without thinking. It has become streamlined and habitual, and is taken over by the unconscious part of your mind. Beyond this stage is *mastery* – but that is another book!

Some gifted learners can go through the middle two conscious stages extremely quickly, taking in skills at an unconscious level. NLP has explored this realm of accelerated learning and we will deal with it more fully later.

Language and physiology

How do you know what neurological level you are dealing with? One way is to listen to the language people use. Here is an example of the same subject at each level: a person is learning psychology.

> *Environment:* It is easy to learn psychology if you have supportive people round you.

> *Behaviour:* I learned that theory.

> *Capability:* I understand what psychology is about.

Beliefs and values: It is important to understand what motivates people.

Identity: I am a psychologist.

You can start to notice the subtle ways that people mark out the level they are on. For example, when someone says, '*I* can't do that', giving the stress to the first word, they are talking about their identity. By contrast, 'I can't do *that*' is about behaviour.

These levels also have broad physiological counterparts. We react to the *environment* with reflexes. *Behaviour* is the actions and thoughts we carry out consciously. *Capabilities* are habitual, semi-conscious or unconscious actions. *Beliefs and values* connect to our autonomic nervous system, such as our heart beat and adrenaline level. Finally, our *identity* at the physiological level is our immune system, that protects us by distinguishing between the self and other. And *beyond identity*? It may involve a balance in the autonomic nervous system between the sympathetic branch that is involved in energizing and stimulating the heart rate, respiration and blood pressure ready for action, and the parasympathetic system which relaxes the same functions. Spiritual writings often speak of acting from a place of stillness (Being), with dynamic purpose, yet having no attachment to the results of that action.

What happens when these levels are confused?

You have probably seen a child make a mistake and an adult say something like, 'Oh, you are stupid.' What is happening? Behaviour has been taken at identity level. Yet to misspell a word or get a sum wrong does not mean someone is a stupid person. The tragedy is that a child often believes it does. This is probably the most common way our self-esteem is undermined. Children are very gifted learners and tend to believe what adults tell them, particularly about their identity. A child who believes he is clumsy, for example, will begin to live out this belief as he grows by being clumsy, not just with plates, but perhaps later with words or cars.

The same pattern can repeat whatever age you are. For example, a salesman loses an order and is told what a useless human being he is by a particularly insensitive manager. Adults are less impressionable and more resilient – sometimes.

The principle here is to give and take criticism at the level of behaviour, not identity. You can still value a person's identity while criticizing his behaviour. This also means he is likely to act on the criticism if it is valid. The positive intention of criticism is to help the person do the best he is capable of.

Have you ever got into an argument like this?

'This house is really untidy.' *(environment)*

'I tidied it this morning!' *(behaviour)*

'Well you didn't do it very well!' *(capability)*

'I did! If you understood how difficult it was, you would be more considerate.' *(belief)*

'Are you calling me inconsiderate?!' *(identity)*

So we have an identity-level crisis in short order from an environmental remark.

One man Ian knows used to get very tense over his work. He had a demanding job as a lawyer. He was forever complaining he did not know how to relax and it started to affect his health. Many people, including a doctor, told him to take a holiday. Now a change in environment might help him to relax in the short term, but it is not going to teach him *how* to relax, which was what he was asking. 'How' is capability. Solutions that only work in the short term are usually on the wrong neurological level.

Changing levels

Knowing these levels is very useful in personal change and personal development work. Change is possible at any level. The question is, which will have the most leverage, that is, give the greatest result for the smallest effort? A change at the belief level is likely to affect skills and behaviour a great deal, a change in identity even more so. You can work from the top down or from the bottom up – all the levels relate together systemically.

A friend of Joseph's was brought up with the belief that he was not a practical person. DIY was replaced by GSTDIFY – Get Someone To Do It For You. In his home, like that of his parents, when something went wrong, you telephoned the local craftsman. Then he bought a new house which needed a lot of work done on it. In this new environment, he had a powerful resource, a stronger belief that linked to his identity: it is foolish to assume you cannot do something until you try it. He did not think he was a foolish person. Two years later, he had rewired the house, decorated every room and built a wardrobe. The old belief lost its hold completely. It was true for him just as long as he had believed it to be so. A change in environment had precipitated a change in belief, behaviour and capability.

To solve a problem at one level it usually helps to go to a different level. A problem cannot be solved with the same level of thinking that created it.

When you are stuck or confused, identify the level you are stuck on:

- You may need more information from the environment.

- You may have all the information, but not know what to do.

- You may know what to do, but not know how to do it.

- You may wonder whether you can do it, whether it is worthwhile and if it conflicts with any of your beliefs and values.

- Or it may not be in keeping with your sense of self.

- Sometimes a person can jump to a still higher level and may even have a spiritual experience, like Saint Paul on the road to Damascus.

Rapport

NLP uses the word *rapport*, as we have seen, to describe a relationship of trust and responsiveness. Rapport is essentially meeting individuals in their model of the world. We all have different upbringings, experiences and ways of being. We are all unique, with different beliefs, capabilities and identities. We all see the world differently. To gain rapport with others you need to acknowledge them and their view of the world. You do not have to agree with it, just recognize and respect it. The question is, how?

Rapport can be established (or broken) at many different levels.

Body language

We build rapport, and therefore trust, in a face-to-face meeting in many ways: with our words, our body language and our voice tone. The words are the most obvious part of any conversation, yet they are only the tip of the communication iceberg. There have been studies, following the classic work by Albert Mehrabian at the University of California at Los Angeles in 1981, of the impact of body language and voice tone on our perception of the trustworthiness of other people. These have shown that if words and body language conflict, we nearly always take the non-verbal message as the more significant, although our conscious attention is mostly on the words. Sometimes we may not know why we do not trust someone; sometimes the conflict is obvious. Would you take lessons in public speaking from someone who mumbled?

Clothes and appearance are also part of our body language. They make a statement about us to the outside world, whether we want them to or not. Our clothes and appearance contribute to the first impressions we make on others. Rapport at this level is partly a matter of credibility. Coming to a business meeting in jeans and trainers (unless you are in California!) is unlikely to gain credibility. People form first impressions quickly, usually in under ten seconds, and tend to stick with them. You never get a second chance to make a first impression.

How can you use your voice and body language to show that you are paying attention to the speaker and respect their model of the world? One of the keys to good relationships is acknowledging others and giving them the attention they deserve. Such acknowledgement brings out the best in us, it is what makes us bloom. Paying attention is an act of acknowledgement which is usually taken at an identity level by the other person.

One way excellent communicators acknowledge others and gain rapport is by matching body language and voice tone with the person they are with. We all do this naturally to some extent. For example, we sit down to talk to someone who is sitting and stand if they are standing. It feels awkward to do otherwise. We observe unspoken rules of personal space and feel uncomfortable if they are breached without permission. We tend to match the amount of eye contact we have with people. It is intimidating to be stared at. On the other hand, if you are comfortable with a lot of eye contact, then you may be put off talking to someone who does not meet your gaze very often.

Matching body language to gain rapport goes further. Next time you are in a restaurant, look round at the people on adjoining tables. Whether they are talking or not, you are likely to know intuitively those who are in rapport. They will tend to have the same general body posture. They may be holding their head at the same angle. There will be a rhythm to the interaction. Couples who are in loving relationships may well be breathing in unison.

If you want to gain rapport with someone, match some aspects of their body language. Adopt a similar posture. Give the same amount of eye contact. Match the speed and general frequency of hand gestures.

The intention behind body matching is to share, and understand to a small extent, the other person's experience of the world. Body matching is a powerful way of entering another person's world because how we use our body influences our emotional state and how we think. Matching is not mimicry, however. Exact copying is not respectful. People quickly notice it and think you are mocking them. Body matching is more like dancing. Dancers do not copy, but complement each other. Their movements express their relationship.

If you doubt the power of rapport by matching body language, try this experiment. Pick a conversation where nothing is at stake and where you feel comfortable about experimenting, then match your companion's body language. Adopt roughly the same body posture and match the frequency and size of their gestures. Notice how well the communication flows. Then mismatch. Change your body language to something quite different. Now notice how well the communication flows. It is likely to change drastically.

Mismatching is the opposite of matching. It is also a useful skill. Do you want a way to extricate yourself from a conversation without appearing rude? Mismatch body language. Looking away or increasing the rate of head nodding are some ways.

Mismatching is disengaging, but it need not invalidate the other person. When Ian was at university, one student he knew liked to give parties, but also liked to go to bed around 3 a.m. So he mismatched in a very obvious way. His parties always finished at about 2 a.m., when he would bring out the vacuum cleaner and under the pretence of cleaning up would vacuum people out of the front door. His parties became famous for the way they finished and lots of people would come for the sheer novelty of the ending.

VOICE

We can also establish rapport with others by matching their voice tone. Again, we do this to some extent without thinking. When your companion is soft spoken, it is natural to moderate your own voice. Voice matching is not mimicry, more like two instruments harmonizing. The easiest way to experiment is to match the volume and the speed of the other person's voice.

Voice matching is a good way of responding to someone who is angry with you. An angry person, whether justified or not, demands your attention. Anger is energy, so it is essential you match the energy and urgency of the person's voice. Match at slightly below their level of volume and speed, not at the same level, or you may escalate into a shouting match. Now, by gradually lowering your own voice, you can lead them into calmer waters. A calm, placating voice tone from the beginning will rarely work because it does not acknowledge the anger and is often interpreted as patronizing.

Matching voice tone is the main way you have of establishing rapport on the telephone. When you want to end a telephone conversation without appearing rude (a very useful skill), mismatch voice tone. Talk faster and louder, while saying the appropriate words of farewell. The caller gets both a verbal and non-verbal message.

Matching body language and voice tone to gain rapport is a good example of NLP taking a pattern that people do naturally, refining it and making it a learnable skill. It is a natural by-product of interest in, and attention on, another person. You can use it consciously to gain rapport, though there are two caveats when you do.

First, you may feel awkward. This is because you are now aware of what you do naturally anyway. You are gaining choice about where and how much you do it. Second, body matching will feel and look hollow and contrived if you use it in an attempt to influence people you have no interest in and do not really want to talk to. Why bother? Just walk away.

Be selective about who you body match. Professionals in contact with people who are physically or mentally ill may use body matching to gain rapport and thus take on some of the unhealthy patterns of the people they treat. This can be a major factor in burn-out and illness in the caring professions. One way round this is to use *cross-over matching*. This is to match another person's body language with a different type of movement, for example tapping your foot in time to their speech rhythm.

WORDS

Your words can also establish rapport. First, using the same technical vocabulary, where appropriate, is one way of establishing professional credibility. Second, people will often mark out words and phrases that are important to them. Using the same words or phrases in your reply shows them you hear and respect their meaning.

Often we paraphrase what people tell us. But although a paraphrase may have the same meaning *to* us, it may not to them. For example, a person might say, 'I just can't *make contact* with my boss.' A reply like 'Oh, you mean you can't communicate with her?' does not acknowledge the important words, and the person may disagree and say of course they can communicate, but they cannot make contact. Sometimes this is very confusing if you do not realize what is happening. NLP takes the words people say very literally and respects their precise meaning for the speaker. We will be saying more about this in Chapter 5.

Body and voice matching creates rapport at the *behaviour* level. If you can consistently create rapport, then you have the *capability* to do it. But body matching is not sufficient for rapport if you mismatch *values*. Rapport built through beliefs and values is strong. Shared beliefs and values establish rapport; political and religious groups are obvious examples. You do not have to share them, simply acknowledge and respect them. Building rapport at this level also means respecting the culture you find yourself in. It may be a foreign culture, a different business culture or a new family culture. The strongest rapport comes from acknowledging the person's *identity*. When a person feels acknowledged at this level, they are open to be influenced.

One person we know has difficulty with his relationships because he is always afraid he is missing something even better. He is charming at parties, but while he is talking to you his eyes are flickering round the room to see if there is anyone else who might be even more interesting. If you have ever tried to have a conversation with a person like this you will know how difficult it is to concentrate on what you are saying. Your thoughts become scrambled, you may get annoyed and start to doubt whether what you are saying is at all interesting. You do not feel acknowledged. This person tends to end up alone at parties. He has lost many real relationships for imaginary ones.

Pacing and leading

Matching body language, voice tonality and words, and respecting beliefs and values, are examples of what NLP calls *pacing*. Pacing is having the flexibility to meet another person in their model of the world, rather than making them come to yours. Imagine walking with a companion, adjusting your own pace to stay with them, rather than insisting they keep up with you. You do not lose your own sense of self or your own values and beliefs in the process. Pacing is not being a psychological cushion – bearing the imprint of the last person to sit on you! In fact you need a strong sense of self to pace others well.

Pacing establishes a bridge. Once you have that, you can lead another person to other possibilities. By matching body language with an angry or upset person, for example, you acknowledge what is important for him, so he no longer needs to insist on the validity of his experience and becomes more available. You then lead him to a calmer state by moderating your voice and changing your posture. You cannot lead without first pacing and gaining rapport.

When Joseph taught the guitar, he met a new student, a little girl of five years old. Her father had brought her for a trial lesson. Although she wanted to learn, she was clearly in awe and very shy. She said hardly a word. All he could do was match her breathing, and the general speed and frequency of her movements as he spoke to her. Gradually he started breathing a little slower. Her breathing calmed and she started to talk a little. Then he used her own words about the guitar and what she wanted to learn, and spoke at the same volume. Gradually her voice became stronger. She opened out. The lesson was a success, when it had looked as if it would be hard going at the start.

Congruence

What would it mean to pace and lead yourself – to be in rapport with yourself? The state of rapport between mind and body is called *congruence* in NLP. Congruence means that you are all of a piece, that your body language, tonality and words carry the same message. Your beliefs and values line up with your actions. You 'walk your talk'. How many body therapists have poor posture? How many doctors do you know who smoke? There are psychiatrists who are difficult to tell apart from their patients!

However, congruence is not perfection. When the gods have a message to deliver, they sometimes choose strange messengers. Congruence is not that all of you is playing exactly the same tune, but all your parts are at least following the same score. If you prefer a visual example, a picture that is all the same colour is not a picture at all. It's a background. You need many different colours to make a complete and interesting picture, including some colours that might look strange on their own. Our weaknesses are our best teachers, pointing us to the most productive ways to learn and change. We can use them to tune the orchestra and refresh the palette, creating richer, fuller symphonies and pictures.

Multiple descriptions

Pacing, as we have seen, is meeting others in their model of the world. This does not mean you lose your own point of view. Central to NLP is an appreciation of the value of having different views of the same event. This is called having a *multiple description*. NLP distinguishes three main points of view (developed mainly by John Grinder from the work of Gregory Bateson):

1. *First position* is your own reality. Think of a time when you were intensely aware of what you thought and believed, regardless of other people. You have just experienced being in first position, regardless of exactly what you thought about.

2. *Second position* is taking another person's point of view. You think, 'How would this appear to them?' Matching body language helps in taking second position. Because communication is an interactive process, the more you can understand how the other person is thinking and feeling, the better you can communicate to get what you both want from the interaction.

3. *Third position* is the ability to take an outside, detached point of view and appreciate the relationship between you and the other. This is an important skill, especially if you are stuck.

Having these three views in a situation is called a *triple description*. All three positions are important and the best communicators move easily between each. A person stuck in first position will be an egotistical dinosaur, blindly trampling the feelings of others. Someone habitually in second position will be too easily influenced, putting others' needs above their own, a martyr neglecting their own needs and well-being. Someone too much in third position will be detached from life, rather than engaging in it fully.

To be able to act wisely you need all three perspectives. They are different, and it is this difference that adds richness and choice. Excitement and creativity come from difference.

Sameness leads to boredom and mediocrity. Multiple description is like looking at all the different-coloured dots arranged in different ways in a stereogram, so the three-dimensional image can emerge. Being able to take multiple perspectives is also part of that general flexibility of response of successful people. The world is always richer than any one view of it. And because this is so, we all take different parts of it and combine them to create our distinctive world. Exactly how we do this is central to NLP.

2

That Is Not What I Meant At All...

Rapport is the first step in good communication. We are all excellent communicators – and still we are misunderstood. If you are a human being you will have been in a situation where you said something you thought was clear, only to be amazed at the response. An innocent remark is taken personally or a well-meant offer of help refused with a reply like 'Don't interfere!' The offer was clear to you but not to the listener. This happens in reverse as well, when what you understood was not what the other person meant. Perhaps someone has said to you, 'It won't take long.' You expect them to be finished in an hour and they were thinking of half a day. Human communication is not like Morse Code where there is a fixed interpretation of each symbol. There is the joke about the two psychoanalysts meeting in the street. One says to the other, 'Good morning. How are you?' And the other thinks, 'I wonder what he meant by that?'

We cannot help making meaning of what we see, hear and feel. We are not only gifted and creative communicators, we are also gifted and creative receivers. Misunderstanding is the price we pay for being able to convey or infer so many subtle shades of meaning. Perhaps the miracle is that we are ever understood at all!

When we communicate, our goal is to transmit meaning. How do we know we have succeeded? When the other person gets that message.

A sender cannot decide what the signal will actually mean to the other person, only what they would like it to mean. There is no such thing as failure in communication – you always succeed in communicating *something*. It just may not be what you intended. The responses you get give you valuable pointers about what to do next. They are your teachers.

One NLP presupposition sums this up:

The meaning of the communication is the response you get.

What would be the consequences of acting as if this NLP presupposition is true?

You might get curious. How are misunderstandings possible? And how can they be prevented? This is usually done by paying attention to the other person's response, rather than mind-reading or wishful thinking. Just by paying attention you could pick up misunderstandings before going miles out of your way and before they have serious consequences.

This is important in business, where managers want to motivate rather than antagonize their colleagues, and where miscommunication about prices and quantities of goods can result in large financial losses. It is important in sales and presentations. One of Joseph's friends in computer sales had thoroughly prepared her script for an important meeting with a client. She knew all about the system and was convinced that as soon as the customer knew what a good system it was, he would buy. All she had to do was tell him. She was a few minutes into her presentation when she noticed the customer's eyes glazing over. It became obvious to her that she was not going to make this sale by continuing. She extricated herself by dropping her papers and, after the confusion of retrieving them, complete with apologies, she said, 'Where were we? Oh yes, what do you want to be able to do with this system?' The customer bought after a good discussion, because he had the opportunity to discover how the system met his needs. By doing something different she was able to regain rapport and achieve her outcome.

The principle is also important in relationships. Have you ever got into an argument and thought, 'Oh no, not again?' It all seems horribly familiar, the same old misunderstanding has come up, the argument seems almost scripted. What would you need to do differently to establish or regain rapport and achieve your outcome?

Modelling excellence is not just about learning from your mistakes. Think back to some of your effective communications, where you got the response you wanted. What did you do that worked? Not just the specific actions you took in that particular instance, but how did you think? Were you right first time? Did you have to adjust? If you were right first time, how did you decide what to do?

When you mean one thing and the other person shows you by their response that they have a different meaning, nobody is wrong and nobody is to blame. Assuming responsibility for your communication does not mean always having to say you are sorry. There is a widespread approach to communication mistakes that concentrates on finding who was to blame, as if finding a scapegoat solves the problem. But no one is to blame for being human. Also, blaming rarely promotes learning. When you do not have to blame yourself or others, you become more open to learning and a sense of wonder. You also become more able to tolerate ambiguity. Faced with a world that is uncomfortably unpredictable, many people become anxious. They want 'yes' or 'no' answers, not 'maybe' and 'perhaps'. But certainty is hard to achieve and the price is usually high. Change is the only thing you can rely on.

The meaning of the communication is what I say it is!

What are the consequences of acting in the opposite way — as if the meaning of your communication is fixed to what you say it is? This is a bewildering world. Other people will still make their own meanings of what you say and misunderstandings will multiply.

There is a nice story of an Arabian wise man who is lost in the desert and sees horsemen in the distance. 'Bandits!' he thinks and, wheeling his own horse, trots in the opposite direction. Looking around, he sees they are following him, so he rides faster.

Five minutes later, they are still gaining on him. He becomes frightened, gallops into a thicket and hides. His pursuers follow him and dismount. He is very relieved to see they are his friends, who were searching for him. They ask him why on earth he is hiding from them behind a bush miles out of the way.

'It's more complicated than you think,' replies the wise man. 'I'm here because of you and you are here because of me.'

Neither was where they wanted to be.

Beyond this bewilderment is an uninviting world of blame, fault and failure. If you believe people *ought* to understand, then it is their fault if they do not. Take the caricature of the loud American abroad who, when faced with blank stares from the native population, simply repeats his instructions s-l-o-w-e-r and LOUDER in the vain hope that this will make them understand.

The same principle applies in reverse. You may blame yourself for misunderstanding. A few gifted individuals manage to both have their cake and eat it — if they do not understand then it's the other person's fault, they should have been clearer; if the other person does not understand then it's still their fault, they are being difficult or obtuse and should have done so! But this is a recipe for anger and frustration.

> 'I'm sure I didn't mean –' Alice was beginning, but the Red Queen interrupted her impatiently.
>
> 'That is just what I complain of! You should have meant! What do you suppose is the use of a child without any meaning? Even a joke should have a meaning – and a child is more important than a joke, I hope. You couldn't deny that, even if you tried with both hands.'
>
> 'I don't deny things with my hands,' Alice objected.
>
> 'Nobody said you did,' said the Red Queen. 'I said you couldn't if you tried.'
>
> *(Lewis Carroll,* Through the Looking Glass*)*

Communication with yourself

What would it mean to act as if the meaning of a communication with yourself were the response you get? It would mean paying attention to the responses you get from your body; your feelings and intuitions.

A colleague of Ian's was setting up an important business deal with some new business partners. He had an immediate, strong feeling on meeting one prospective partner that the man was not to be trusted. He did not understand how or why, but he became very uncomfortable about going through with the deal. He pulled out, fortunately, for the whole enterprise was mismanaged and collapsed in a short time. This colleague acted on the response he got – he did not try to discount it or tell himself he should not feel like that.

As well as giving us intuitions, our bodies may respond to our lifestyle by becoming ill. A combination of late nights, lack of sleep, overwork and skipped meals will often provoke this response. Acting on it would mean taking care of ourselves and changing our lifestyle. When we continually ignore our own needs because we think we 'ought' to be able to cope, or someone else tells us we should, our body will respond, sooner or later, with pain or illness.

Exploring relationships

A relationship is two people eliciting responses from each other. If you want a change in response, then you must change your own actions. This will change the meaning for the other person and the spell is broken. Most of us have a relationship where we think, 'If only that person would stop acting that way, then everything would be fine.' It may be a family member or a work colleague. Think of a relationship like that if you have one, to explore further.

What do you think it is about their behaviour that is the problem? For example, you may feel they are aggressive, insensitive or fault finding, so you may feel browbeaten, angry or irritated. Label both your own and the other person's behaviour. You might wonder at which logical level you are threatened. Is this an identity issue for you? One that challenges your beliefs and values? Even thinking about this relationship can put you into an unresourceful state. You do not want to carry that into what you do next, so now think of something different. Move, shake off that feeling. In NLP this is called *changing state*.

Second, imagine what the relationship is like from the other person's point of view. This is going to second position. How do they experience your behaviour? What sort of label would they put on it? How do they feel? Shake off that emotional state before continuing.

Now, go outside the relationship, become a detached observer. This is going to third position. A good way to do this is to imagine a stage in front of you. See both of you on stage. See that other person doing what they do. See yourself responding to them.

Shift your question from 'How can I change that person's behaviour?' to 'How am I reinforcing or triggering that person's behaviour?'

How else could you respond to him or her? What prompts you to continue doing what you do in this relationship?

When you communicate you are seeking to influence another person; you have an outcome in mind. Deciding what you want is the second pillar of NLP and the subject of the next chapter.

3

The Ultimate Question

What is the ultimate question?

For many people it is: 'What is the meaning of life?', 'Is there a God?' or 'Why are we here?' Those are important questions. But we have another that you need to answer before any of the preceding ones make sense.

The reason you ask questions at all is because you want to know the answers. You want something.

So we suggest as the ultimate question:

What do you want?

Everything we do has a reason behind it. We always want something, although we are not always clear what it is. This applies right down to the most mundane levels. When you are hungry, your goal is to eat; when you are tired, your goal is to sleep. The streets are full of people, walking, driving, catching buses, trains and aeroplanes, all going somewhere for a reason. Were this not so, human behaviour would be random and incomprehensible.

So the presupposition of NLP is:

Human behaviour is purposeful.

What do you want right now? You are reading this book, so you want to understand NLP, be entertained and explore some new ideas. You may be reading for relaxation. From a wider view, you have hopes and dreams you want to fulfil. You have long-term and short-term goals, those things you want and need: possessions, skills, work, relationships, states of mind, ways of working or being. NLP calls these *outcomes* — results that you want to create in the world. An outcome is much more specific than a goal. You only have an outcome when you know what you will see, hear and feel when you have it. Goals are what you want. Outcomes are what you create. As it is, you are creating results in your life all the time, even when you do nothing; the only question is, are they the results you want? We all know you don't always get what you want, sometimes due to events beyond your control, sometimes because you do not plan thoroughly enough, but if you do not know what you want, you have no chance of getting it. Setting outcomes is the key to becoming the dominant creative force in your life. It is a way of thinking, not just an occasional activity at New Year. If you do not set outcomes then either chance or other people will determine what you get.

When you set outcomes for yourself, do not be limited by what you consider to be currently possible. There will be many things in your life that seemed impossible when you first considered them, yet now you can look back with satisfaction at how you actually did achieve them.

So you can have whatever outcomes you wish, just notice if they seem possible at the present moment. We create our future every day when we decide what we want.

Some people do not set outcomes, usually for one of two reasons. Either they are afraid of taking a risk, making a mistake and wasting time and effort. Or they are afraid of losing their freedom and spontaneity. Both these reactions are reasonable but self-limiting.

A better way is to give yourself permission to change or discard an outcome if appropriate in the face of feedback. Know what you want, be sensitive to what you are getting and change what you do as necessary.

The question 'What do you want?' generates outcomes that move you towards a solution, a desired state. The common question 'What's the problem?' focuses on what is wrong in the present state and, of itself, does not move you forward. Focusing on the problem generates questions like 'Why do I have this problem?', 'How does it limit me?' and 'Who is to blame?' Finding the historical reasons for a problem and allocating blame do not provide a way out of the impasse.

Outcomes

We fail to achieve our outcomes for three main reasons:

1. They may not be realistically achievable.

2. They may be insufficiently motivating.

3. Although they are desired, they may not be desirable from a wider viewpoint.

To turn a goal into an outcome, to make it realistic, achievable, motivating and desirable, you have to explore it from different points of view.

Make sure it is expressed in the positive

This means moving towards what you want, not away from what you do not want. Having a negative outcome is like going shopping with a list of what you are not going to buy. What are two common and difficult goals? To lose weight and to give up smoking. One of the reasons they are so difficult is that they are both expressed in the negative. Any goal that has the words 'lose' or 'give up' or 'don't want' is not expressed in the positive. Why are goals expressed in the negative hard to achieve? Try this negative goal: do not think about your next-door neighbour. Whatever you do, do not let any idea about your next-door neighbour come into your mind. What goes through your mind in response to this? In order not to think about your neighbour, you have to think about them, so you know what not to think about. You have to keep in mind what not to do, which means you are doing it. Now think of your family. That is easy and, when you do, you will automatically forget your neighbour.

To turn a negative outcome into a positive, ask, 'What would this goal do for me if I got it?' or 'What do I want instead?' For example, 'giving up smoking' may become 'having healthy lungs', 'being healthier, fitter' or 'having more money'.

Determine what you have to do and what others have to do

Have as much of the outcome under your direct control as possible. If others need to act for you, think how you can arrange a 'win–win outcome' – so they get something that is important to them at the same time. We can achieve little without others, and unless you think out the consequences for them from their viewpoint so they win as well as you, they may only help you once, if at all. Ask yourself, 'What is it I need to do to ensure these others *want* to help me achieve my outcome?'

Make the outcome as specific as possible

Imagine it in as much detail as you can. How long will it take? Set a realistic time limit, with an exact date if possible. Some outcomes you will want *within* the deadline, others *at* the deadline. If your outcome is to be promoted at work, then a promotion next week could catch you unprepared to shoulder the responsibility immediately. Where and when do you want this goal? In which places, situations or parts of your life do you want it? Where would you not want it? For example, you might set an outcome to be more relaxed about spending money, buying gifts and eating out only during your holiday. Once the holiday is over, you may want a different kind of spending pattern. With whom do you want the goal and with whom do you not want it? For example, an outcome to be more playful would be good with your children, but you might think twice about applying it with your boss. The more you can make your outcome specific, the more real it becomes and the more you will notice opportunities to achieve it.

Be clear about your evidence for achievement

How will you know you have achieved your outcome? This is a really important question. Unless you can see the finishing line, you will never know if the race is over. The evidence will be through your five senses. What exactly will you see? What exactly will you hear? What exactly will you feel? What is the very last piece of evidence before you get the outcome? For example, evidence for being more healthy might be that you have a small waist, and you wake up feeling alert and breathing easily instead of coughing. You will be the correct weight for your height, your complexion will have improved and at least one friend will tell you that you look better than before.

You cannot achieve an outcome, or learn anything, without feedback, and the sooner the feedback comes the better. For example, you are learning a foreign language. You do a test one week and you get the results a week later. By the time you get the feedback you have forgotten the original test and meanwhile continue to make the same mistakes. The longer the time between action and feedback, the harder it is to learn and adjust what you are doing. In relationships, this feedback comes down to good communication between partners, avoiding that *cri de coeur*, 'Why didn't you tell me before?'

Consider the resources you have or can create to achieve this outcome

Obvious resources are money and material possessions that you can use directly. People are resources. They may be able to help you directly or you can use them as role models. If you know of someone who has achieved a similar outcome, then you may be able to ask them how they did it. You can also use historical characters or fictional characters from books, films or television as role models. All that is needed is that they faced a similar challenge and overcame it.

Personal qualities and skills are also resources. For example, perseverance, networking ability and rapport skills may be a help. If there are qualities you need and do not yet have, think about how you could develop them. It might be through training, role models or accessing and developing those qualities in yourself (self-modelling). You will be able to transfer qualities from one part of your life to another. It is worth writing a list of your resources. You may not need them all, but the more choices you have, the more likely you are to get your outcome, and it is heartening to look down a list of helpful people, skills and possessions.

Consider the consequences and by-products of achieving your outcome

George Bernard Shaw once said that there are two tragedies in life. One is not to get your heart's desire. The other is to get it. He was no doubt thinking of all the other things that may come with your heart's desire that you did not wish for. In the myth, King Midas wished that everything he touched turned to gold. And so it did, including his friends, loved ones, food and drink.

Think of your outcome from different points of view. One of the best ways to explore the consequences is to take second position with significant other people. How does your outcome appear from their point of view? How does it affect them? How do they feel about it? When you think like this you will gain their trust and they will help you more.

What else would happen? What will you have to sacrifice? For example, suppose your outcome is to move house. Other issues might be: what access do you have to shops? How far away from your friends will you be? Will you still be able to see them? What are the new local amenities like? How easy is the journey to work? How good are the local schools?

What will you have to give up by getting what you want? A promotion at work could bring a change of boss, longer working hours and a changed relationship with co-workers. Also think about the time, money and the effort, both mental and physical, you will need to invest. Is the goal worth it?

Recognize the positive by-products of your present behaviour

Invariably the present situation will have some good qualities. If it had none at all, you would have changed things already. How can you incorporate them into your outcome, so that you keep what is good about your present circumstances?

How does your outcome relate to your larger plans?

Your outcome is likely to be part of a larger outcome. Relate it to your other plans and outcomes that are important to you. What does it help to achieve and why is this important?

When you connect your outcome to your values and life plans, it will be motivating. It is difficult to commit to an outcome that seems unimportant and disconnected from the rest of your life.

What smaller outcomes may be part of this outcome?

Your outcome may be large and unwieldy as it stands. There may be obstacles. You may need to break it down into a series of smaller, more manageable outcomes. Decide on the right sequence in which to do them, then begin.

Lastly, does this outcome feel right to you?

Is it congruent with your sense of self, your identity? Is it *you?* If it is, take your insights and form an action plan, including one thing you can do immediately. Unless you act, the outcome will remain a dream. There is software available that will take you through these questions to refine your outcome.

Outcome checklist

- Is it expressed in the positive, moving towards something you want, rather than away from something you do not want?

- Can you start and maintain this outcome? What will you have to do and what will others have to do? How can you persuade them to help you?

- Is the outcome specific? Do you have a clear idea of when, where and with whom you want the outcome?

- What is your sensory evidence that you have achieved the outcome? What will you see, hear and feel?

- What resources do you have to help you achieve this outcome? List your possessions, money, people, role models, skills and personal qualities.

- What are the wider consequences of achieving your outcome? What will you have to give up? How will others be affected? What money and mental and physical effort will you have to put in? Is it worth it?

- How can you incorporate the good things about the present situation into the outcome?

- What larger outcome is this part of?

- Do you need to set smaller, supporting outcomes? Are there obstacles?

- Is it *you*?

- Act!

Resources and self-modelling

An outcome takes you from a present state that is unsatisfactory to a desired state. Some people focus more on the *present state* and what is wrong with it, others on the *desired state* and the anticipated rewards.

To move from one to the other you need resources. We already have the resources we need. We are all models of excellence at least some of the time and with NLP you can get access to these resources. The more you find inside, the less you need to go outside. You have power – once you start using NLP you are finished with being a victim. You do not need to go outside yourself for answers, and the realization that you are capable means that envy makes no sense. To harvest your resources, think about what is working in your life and what has worked. At the end of each day, remember what you did well and start to form a collection of resources that will be easy to think back to.

Joseph was working with a very good tennis player who had been to a number of coaches and psychologists. Coaching is important when it concentrates on reinforcing good habits rather than drawing attention to bad ones. However, the coaches had done the opposite. The player knew exactly what he was doing wrong and was constantly on the lookout for mistakes in his game. The advice had paralysed him.

Joseph started to work with him to recall the many times in the past when he had played really well and everything had gone *right*, using the word 'focus' to associate with that state. At the highest levels of professional sport it is concentration and mental skills that make the difference. This focused state cannot be achieved through conscious trying or analysis. The moment you 'try' to do something, you are not doing it. Now, instead of trying to avoid mistakes, the player modelled his own states of excellence and so was able to enter them more easily and more often. His results improved tremendously. He started to do himself justice.

Self-modelling starts with an outcome:

You ask yourself, 'What do you want?'

The next question is, 'When have you had it?' (It can be in any context.)

When you have an instance, however slight, ask, 'What did you do that worked?'

Remember as exactly as possible. How were you thinking and what actions did you take? What did you believe then? Beliefs are really important in self-modelling; they can block or release excellence. What beliefs were you enacting? They were probably permissive ones, like 'this is possible', 'this is easy', 'this is important' or 'I deserve to succeed'. When you did have the resource you want now, what was the effect on you? Did you enjoy it? Was it liberating? What was the effect on others? Were they pleased? Frightened? Uncomprehending?

What could be significant about the experience you are remembering? There may be a special reason why it stays in your mind. The circumstances may have been unusual, you may have surprised yourself or someone else may have made a significant contribution. Whatever it was, it can help you recreate a similar situation to make the resource more easy to access.

Finally what was the learning in this experience? What conclusions did you draw and are they still valid?

Self-modelling can help you to get your outcome directly or help you get the resources you need. Once you know your outcome, keep it steady and change your behaviour until you get it or the feedback tells you that this outcome is wrong for you. If what you are doing is not working, do something different. Individuals with the most flexibility have the best chance of achieving what they want.

Congruence and incongruence

When you set an outcome, you are working to change your life from how it is now to something you prefer. You move from a *present state* to a *desired state*. Sometimes the change is easy and sometimes it is not. Sometimes we are *congruent* – fully committed to the change, in rapport with ourselves. Other times we are *incongruent* – at odds with ourselves, with internal conflict.

This conflict can happen in two ways. Incongruence can be *simultaneous*, when we try to do two different things at once. For example, you have probably been in the situation where someone asks you to do them a favour that takes you out of your way. You want to please them. And you want to get on with what you are doing. So you may say, 'Yes,' but your body and voice tone say, 'No.' Your 'yes' is really a 'yes, but…' Another example is when you are trying to finish some work, and somehow your mind keeps wandering off the task. One part of you wants to complete the task, the other wants time off, and they both want it now!

It is uncomfortable to be on the receiving end of this sort of incongruence, especially for children. Perhaps when you were young you did something you were proud of, maybe a drawing or a painting. You showed it excitedly to an adult who said 'Yes, very nice' in a bored or sneering tone of voice. As a child, do you remember the feeling of confusion and disquiet? It is easier to deal with straightforward rejection – at least you know where you are. Incongruence gives you a mixed message. Which one do you act on? Children who are surrounded by incongruent adults become very unsure of themselves, whereas really it is the adults' responses they are unsure of, and rightly so.

To deal resourcefully with the incongruence of others, you need to recognize it for what it is. This makes it understandable. You may then want to challenge it by saying something like, 'I noticed you said "Yes", but you also seemed to have some reservations. Will you tell me what they are?' It is especially important for salespeople to surface incongruence in customers, as it hides objections to the product that need to be dealt with.

The second type of incongruence is *sequential*. You do something and then you wish you hadn't. The first 'you' is somehow different from the second 'you'. You meet this type of incongruence from others when they promise they will do something and then don't.

We are made up of many different parts, like a team that sometimes pulls together and other times in different directions or like an orchestra that sometimes plays in tune and sometimes not. We are not the same person to everyone we meet. Think how differently you behave towards your friends at a party, towards a policeman that stops you for a traffic offence and towards young children. A different part of us comes into play for each different situation. We do not have a monolithic personality structure, yet we do have a sense of unity about these different parts – they are in one team, they do belong to one orchestra. You are not your behaviour. You are not any one team member or any one instrumentalist in the orchestra. When the team pulls together and the orchestra plays in tune, you are congruent.

Conscious and unconscious

Congruence is not an all or nothing state – sometimes we are more congruent than others and many times we do not know why we are incongruent. Sometimes we just do not understand what possessed us to do something. We were 'beside our selves'. NLP, in common with nearly all psychology, makes a fundamental distinction between the part of us that is self-aware and aware of the world – the conscious mind – and the part that is not – the unconscious mind. Our conscious mind makes decisions, thinks, analyses, sets directions, decides what to do and acts as if it is in control. It is like a searchlight. It shines the light of reason and analysis on the vast darkness that surrounds us and sees only what is in the light. It may believe that what it can see is all that exists. But according to classical studies in psychology, we can only pay conscious attention to between five and nine pieces of information at any one time. To experience this for yourself, pay attention to reading this book, and while you do that be aware of the sounds around you, as well as the feeling in your left foot, the taste in your mouth and the feel of the book in your hands, your breathing, your heart beat... Very soon you will sense your conscious limits.

The unconscious mind has a far greater influence and can accomplish far more than the conscious. Think how tortuous and slow it would be if you had to think consciously of how to walk, how to talk, how to write. You do not give a conscious command to each muscle group to accomplish these tasks, it is all dealt with by your unconscious. Learning and change always take place at the unconscious level. Then we become aware of the change and integrate it into our lives.

The conscious mind has reasons and insights, but is powerless to change on its own. Think of a change you would like to make in your life. If it were a matter of conscious will-power, you would have made it already. It is not, yet we often berate and punish ourselves for not having the will-power to change.

Joseph used to smoke cigarettes quite heavily. He 'tried' to give up on many occasions using will-power. He knew it was unhealthy and a waste of money, but these arguments never seemed to apply to the next cigarette. Then he met his future wife. She did not smoke and had no intention of starting. She said very little about his smoking and did not try to persuade him to give up, yet he stopped smoking for good within a few days. It was very easy – no will-power was involved.

Behaviour and intention

Our unconscious controls most of our behaviour, whether we understand its purpose consciously or not. To understand our deeper motives, we need to build a bridge between the conscious and unconscious. Congruence comes from rapport between the two. Sometimes we find what we do incomprehensible from a conscious viewpoint, yet there will be a good reason. Our unconscious supports us 24 hours a day. We never forget to breathe, our heart never forgets to beat.

There are two of the most important presuppositions in NLP here:

The unconscious mind is benevolent.

All behaviour has a positive intention.

Our behaviour is always trying to achieve something valuable for us. What appears as negative behaviour is only so because we do not see the purpose. Even suicide can have a positive intention. People who have tried to commit suicide, which seems to be the ultimate self-destruction, give reasons that make sense once you understand their world: to be at peace or to escape the pain they live with.

How do you find out the positive intention behind something? Ask a very simple question and continue asking it until you get an answer: 'What does that behaviour get for you?' In this way you make a distinction between the ends and the means. The end, the purpose, is valuable. The means, the behaviour, need not be.

Once you act as if this were true, you can begin to trust yourself, to be your own best friend – even in the moments when you seem to be your own worst enemy. You can begin to accept yourself and that is the first step in personal change. If you do not acknowledge what is there, you cannot change it.

What you can do is pace your own incongruence, your own different parts, just as you would people at a meeting who are violently disagreeing. When you can pace different parts of yourself, you will get more in rapport with yourself and be more settled and have a clearer sense of self. You can begin to be curious about your behaviour. How interesting! How strange! What is the purpose of that? You can also begin to understand other people and realize that if you were in their shoes, with their beliefs and values, carrying their past experience, in their emotional state, you would act no differently.

Self-acceptance and forgiveness are natural – they need not be another set of virtues that we may struggle to live up to. They are not 'being good'. They are the only rational response to this incredibly fascinating and unpredictable world we are in. When we can forgive ourselves then we can forgive others. Truly to know all is to forgive all.

This does not mean there is no morality and everything is permissible. It does not mean there is no right and wrong. Behaviour can be abominable. Human beings are capable of cruel and terrible acts, and such acts need to be stopped or prevented. But even the behaviour of a mass murderer has a positive intention from their point of view, although they may not know it consciously. From your point of view, or society's point of view, it is hurtful and must be stopped. But you can still honour the intention behind the behaviour and see that there is a human being behind that behaviour. Honour the intention and change the behaviour.

Many attempts at change, both personal and organizational, work only in the short term. This is usually because the intention behind the behaviour has not been satisfied. So it expresses itself in another way and you find yourself chasing symptoms. In that case, go back to asking yourself what that behaviour gets for you.

Signals from the deep

If we presuppose the unconscious is benevolent we can start to mine its incredible resources and look within ourselves for strength. The unconscious can be a friend. How do you establish rapport with it? By mutual respect and trust, and paying attention to the messages it gives you.

What are the signals of the unconscious? First, any habit or behaviour that clashes badly with your normal character shows there is a part of you that has not been acknowledged. Especially if it is repetitive. The unconscious balances the conscious, so your out-of-character behaviour shows there is an important intention that the conscious mind is neglecting. To vow not to do it again does not work, for the part that makes the vow is not the part that does the behaviour.

Pain and illness are another signal. When you are ill with a cold or flu, the positive intention of those symptoms is to heal the body, while the positive intention of pain is to alert you to the fact that something is wrong and you need to take action.

A stress headache is another example. For many people, the first impulse is to reach for an aspirin in the medicine cabinet. This may suppress the pain, but a pill will teach you nothing about avoiding the stress in future. Often pain killers make no difference to stress headaches anyway. The headache is a signal, and the more you try to ignore it, the worse it is likely to become, like a child clamouring for attention. The headache often eases when you start to pay attention to it and ask, 'What are you trying to tell me?' This approach is no substitute for medical attention where it is needed, but it can work very well with many psychosomatic ailments.

Ian found that he was developing toothache one Monday. Toothache is a signal that cannot be ignored, it tells you in no uncertain terms your tooth needs attention. He had an extremely busy few days ahead and it was very difficult to take time to visit the dentist. There were two obvious choices – take pain killers or go to the dentist. He chose a third. He paid attention to his experience. It seemed the pain was more like a warning, so he negotiated with it. He thanked his unconscious for the signal, for without it he would not know the tooth needed attention. He acknowledged the signal and proposed a deal. If it was appropriate for the unconscious to stop the signal and remove the pain, so he could do his work, he promised he would go to the dentist and give the tooth proper attention at the end of the week. If the tooth needed attention immediately, he asked for the signal, that is, the pain, to continue for the rest of the morning and he would book an emergency dental appointment immediately. The pain stopped within half an hour. He was able to do his work during the week without problem. And he kept his promise and went to the dentist at the end of the week.

We live in a culture that is fearful of inner experience which is not immediately gratifying. Yet this is information and tells us we need to make some change. Information is the lifeblood of any organization, from a multinational business down to the human body.

Pacing yourself: congruence signal

Paying attention to your experience, whatever it is, brings your conscious and unconscious into rapport. You begin to *calibrate* your own experience – to know what you are feeling and what it means. You become sensitive to your own body. You are then pacing yourself and it becomes easier to lead yourself to places you want to go but have not got to yet. You will find you become more relaxed and intuitive. Intuition is insight without awareness of the steps that led up to it.

To establish this rapport you need to notice the more subtle, quieter signals from the unconscious. First establish your signal for congruence, when you know you can count on support from all the parts within you:

- Start by becoming aware of all the internal pictures, voices, sounds and feelings that are 'normal' for you. Then change state by moving and thinking of something else.

- Think of a time in the past when you were congruent, fully committed to doing something. It does not matter what it was – something mundane will work perfectly well.

- Now pay attention to that experience as you associate back into that state of congruence. What is it like? Be aware of your internal sounds, pictures and feelings.

- When you have a good taste of that state, come out of it and change state. Do this for three examples of congruence.

- Identify some part that was present in all of those experiences that you intuitively think is absolutely characteristic of those states of congruence. It may be a feeling in your body or a particular voice tone or a picture. It must be involuntary, so either you cannot produce it consciously at all or you can tell the difference between when you produce it consciously and when it spontaneously arises as a congruence signal.

- Make a test. Try to produce that key characteristic without accessing the congruence state. If you can, go back and take another part of the experience and test that. When you cannot, you have got your congruence signal.

This signal will be present in all your congruent states. This gives you a signal for congruence that you cannot consciously fake. It may be an all-or-nothing signal, or it may be gradual, so you can tell by the strength of the signal how much support you have from your unconscious. Use this signal when you are contemplating a decision or project to find out how much support you have and therefore how successful you are likely to be.

Find out your signal for incongruence in a similar way. Select three times when you remember you were in at least two minds over a decision and identify a sound, picture or feeling that is important and you cannot consciously reproduce. This is your incongruence signal; it may be a graded signal that lets you know just how incongruent you are.

These signals can be two of your best friends.

Personal change

- Change is *easy* if... It is safe, you keep the positive by-products of your present state and you allow the unconscious to make it.

- Change is *hard* if... It is risky, you do not find another way to fulfil the purpose of the present behaviour and you 'try' to do it consciously.

4

Getting in a State

States

A state is your way of being at any moment; the sum of your thoughts, feelings, emotions, and mental and physical energy. States vary in intensity, length and familiarity. Some have names, for example love, fascination, alertness, anger, jealousy, fatigue or excitement, while others are less easy to pin down – we may feel in a 'good mood' or a 'bad mood' or just 'out of sorts'. How is this possible?

Once we start to look at the structure of our experience we can discover how we move in and out of different states, and choose which we want to move into and which ones to avoid. Many states are highly valued and greatly sought after: love, happiness, health, ecstasy, the feeling of being accepted, of feeling safe. We spend time, money and effort looking for these states outside ourselves. Money is often pursued as an end in itself, yet it is no more than a means to attain these states. Few people given a choice between riches and good health would choose riches.

The state you are in is very important. It affects your health, the quality of your decisions, how well you learn and how successfully you carry out a task. Would you want to make important decisions while feeling ill, with a temperature of 102°, after a sleepless night?

We remember the very high and very low states. When we are in a very good state, it is great to be alive. When we are down, events we normally shrug off can seem overwhelming. It is not an experience itself, but how we react to it, that gives our quality of life. How we react depends on our state.

We do not spend most of our life at the peaks or in the depths, but in the places between the two. Stop for a moment and make a list of the states you have experienced today. Give them names if they have none. You will find that what seems to be even ground at first glance is actually very varied. Our states change all the time. Trying to hang on to them is like gripping a handful of water in the vain hope it will not slip through your fingers. How do states change, what can you do about it and how could you use and enhance what happens naturally? How much choice do we have about how we feel?

Everyone knows we respond to outside events, becoming angry, excited, loving or exasperated in response to other people and situations. But not so many realize that we can change our state *at will*. This has far-reaching implications for how we learn, how we affect others and how successful we are in the world.

The next two NLP principles go together:

Having choice is better than not having choice.

People make the best choice they can at the time.

When you have choice about your state, you have more emotional freedom. The choices people make are limited by the states they find themselves in. When we increase the range of choice – and emotional freedom – we will have more, perhaps better, choices. There are no unresourceful people, only unresourceful states.

If you want to change your present state, the first thing is to become aware of it, for you cannot deliberately change a state while you remain unaware of it. Start from where you are. Explore the state you are in at the moment. Give it a name. Be aware of your body. Notice the feelings you have in the different parts of your body. If you are uncomfortable, change position. Now be aware of any mental pictures you might have. Do not try to change them. Become aware of any internal voices or sounds. How much mental and physical space do you have? Get a sense of your boundaries. Now you have turned the spotlight of consciousness on your state, notice how it has changed.

To try to solve a problem in the stuck state brought on by wrestling with that problem is futile. A bath of very hot water is not a problem unless you are in it. Rather than think of all the ways you could cool the water down, get out first!

Your baseline state

Some states you 'visit' more than others and there are a small number that you return to regularly. Of these, one will be your *baseline state*, that familiar state where you feel most at home. Is your home a comfortable and well-furnished one? If it had a name, what would it be? Is your baseline state balanced and harmonious or do you habitually feel unbalanced and incongruent? What do you like about it and what would you add if you could?

When your baseline state is long established, it can seem the only way to be, instead of only one way to be. If you are uncomfortable in your baseline state, remember you can change it like any other and custom design one that is a pleasure to return to.

Think of your baseline state from four points of view:

1. *Your physiology:* the state of your body. How healthy, comfortable and balanced is it? Do you have a characteristic posture? If an artist were to draw a caricature of you, what points would they bring out? What is your energy level? How is it shown in the

way you walk, the way you stand and the way you sit? How light or heavy does your body feel?

2. *Your thoughts:* your level of attention, awareness and mental energy. Are you most aware of your mental pictures, words or feelings?

3. *Your predominant emotion.* Is it happy, sad, angry?

4. *Your spiritual state.* How do you relate to something larger than yourself, however you may think about it – God, spirit, energy or the rest of mankind?

Look at your state in terms of logical levels. How do the environments you choose contribute to your state, for good or ill? What do you do that reinforces or takes you out of this state? How do your skills fit with this state? Your beliefs and values will have a tremendous influence on your baseline state. And do you think of your baseline state as part of your identity?

Here are some other questions to ponder about your baseline state.

- Where does it come from?

- Can you trace it back to a particular incident or a particular decision?

- Have you had it as long as you can remember or is it a more recent acquisition?

- Have you modelled it on somebody or is it all your own work?

- Did you learn it, perhaps from your parents or some significant person in your early life?

- Did you learn it consciously or unconsciously?

We take beliefs and values, behaviour and capabilities from our parents, and we often take the state that goes with them.

Learning state

The phenomenon of 'state-dependent learning' is well known: to remember what you have learned, you have to regain the state you were in when you learned it. Actually this is only one narrow aspect of a wider principle: all learning is state dependent. How well you learn depends on the state you are in at the time.

What state enables you to learn quickly, easily and enjoyably? How often were you in that state in your formal education? This is an obvious question, yet most attention in formal education still goes on the curriculum, the books and resources and teaching methods rather than the learner. There seems to be a built-in assumption that if you get the curriculum and the teaching methods right then miraculously people will learn whatever they are taught. Tell that to a teacher taking a class of resistant adolescents, all of whom would rather be somewhere else!

When you want to learn something, the first question to ask yourself is, 'What state do I want to be in to learn this?' Good learners have a set of learning strategies and, more important, they manage their state, because without a good state, the strategies are not available. You have probably been under test at some time in your life, for example school examinations, a sports event, public speaking or having a job interview. However carefully you prepare, anxiety can wreck your state and spoil your chances, and suddenly you can't remember all those things you were going to say. But if you can manage your 'performance state', then the rest will follow.

When you want to teach something, whether you are an educator, trainer, teacher or presenter, ask yourself how you can elicit a learning state in your audience. You may have been lucky enough to have had a teacher at school who made their subject interesting. How did they do it? Usually by bringing enthusiasm and commitment to the subject. States are contagious, so their fascination and involvement made it fascinating and involving for others. The best way to get someone in a learning state is to enter that state yourself.

Another way to elicit a state is to tell a story. If you want people to be curious, tell them a mysterious story. It need have nothing at all to do with the subject you are teaching. Once they are curious, then you can move on to other material.

The principle of pacing and leading applies – you will need to pace the initial state of your audience, especially if they are resistant. Once you have paced and have rapport, you can lead them into a more appropriate state. Sometimes to go straight to a learning state is too big a jump, so you will have to change their state to a neutral one before leading them into a learning state. Changing physiology changes state, so you could, say, get the group up and moving on a structured or informal task.

Noticing states

We elicit states in others all the time through our words, voice tone and body language, often without knowing what we are doing, but we often either do not notice or ignore another person's state. *Calibration* is the NLP term for the skill of recognizing states in others. How can we do this? We cannot always rely on others telling you how they feel and sometimes our calibration skills are so poor that we only notice someone is upset when they burst into tears! However, there are many subtle indicators of a person's state: their breathing rate and depth, skin colour, head angle, facial muscles, voice tone and pupil dilation. All these things are sensory specific and do not involve any guesswork. All you have to do is pay attention to them.

NLP does not hold with universal body language signs that always go with a particular state; crossing your arms does not always mean you are defensive, and touching your hair does not mean you are lying. This is the 'dream dictionary' school of psychology where gestures have fixed meanings and can be interpreted by rote. You would have to pay attention to a particular person and notice that every time they lied they also touched their hair, before you could make a valid deduction. In this, as in other NLP generalizations, the answer is in the person you are with, not in the generalization.

Calibration is not mind-reading, it is correlating signs you can see and hear with the other person's state. Our senses are extraordinary and acute; we are capable of picking up much more than we habitually do.

Try this experiment with a friend. Ask your friend to think of a person they like very much. As they do this, take a mental snapshot of them, particularly their face, and notice their breathing rate, muscle tone, skin colour, size of lips, posture and angle of the head. Ask them to count up to three so you can hear their voice tone. Pay attention to these signs that you normally disregard – they are the physiology of your friend's state.

Now ask your friend to think of someone they dislike, and notice how they look and sound different. Next, ask them to think of one of the two people without telling you which one.

You will know which it is simply by calibrating which physiology they go into.

Anchors

The two most important questions so far are 'What state do I want to be in to make best use of what is happening to me?' and then 'How can I arrange it?'

Our states are constantly changing as we react to the environment. To have choice about your state, you need to know what triggers it. Think of television advertisements. The most effective are those that link a product to a desirable state. For example, many car advertisements say nothing about the car except the name and manufacturer; what they do is set a scene that associates the car with some desirable state like excitement, feeling free, being in control or successful. Buy this car, they say, and you buy this state. Television advertisements are all the more effective because they are repeated many times to viewers who are in a light 'TV trance' with their critical faculties suspended.

The sight and sound of certain things will change your state, for example police sirens, that special piece of music, a plate of your favourite food, the smell of tar on the road, chocolate. NLP calls any stimulus that changes our state an *anchor*. An anchor may be visual, like the sight of a newborn baby or holiday photographs. It may be auditory, like an advertising jingle, or kinaesthetic, like a handshake or a relaxing massage. It may be olfactory, like the smell of roses or boiled cabbage, or gustatory – a particular taste that evokes a specific feeling or memory. It may be external, in the environment, or internal, within the mind, and it can operate at every logical level – for example, your name is an anchor for your identity, and religious symbols are anchors for beliefs and values. Mascots are anchors. Many professional athletes have a particular warming-up routine, a ritual that they will use every time they compete. This is their anchor for a peak performance – it gets them into that state of focus and readiness for competition. Rituals, including, perhaps especially, religious rituals, can be regarded as anchors for achieving certain state changes. Words are also anchors. In this book we want to anchor 'NLP' to a state of curiosity, even fascination, about yourself and others.

Anchors are universal. What makes them universal is our human ability to link stimulus to response without thinking, so you do not have to evaluate every stimulus you receive. Do you evaluate a red traffic light every time you see one?

We consciously choose very few of our anchors – they have been built up randomly throughout our lives. Many of them are neutral and some trigger unresourceful states. Many anchors are linked to the past and may be out-of-date. They are like fossils that never get properly examined. Perhaps one of your parents or teachers used a particular voice tone, and when you heard it, you just knew you were in trouble. That same voice tone may still have the power to make you feel defensive, whoever uses it. You may not even remember the power of the original voice. Anchors have an effect whether we are aware of them or not.

The first practical step is to become aware of the anchors that put you in an unresourceful state. Once you know them, you can choose whether or not to respond. Many spiritual disciplines talk of that moment of choice before reacting. The more you can enter that moment, the easier it becomes.

The second step is to design your own anchors. A business acquaintance of ours has a number of pictures and photographs on the wall of his office. One he deliberately hung upside down. Whenever he sees it, it reminds him that there are other ways of looking at issues besides the obvious one.

What sort of anchor are you?

What states do you elicit in others and are they what you want? As we have seen, you cannot not communicate, so you are bound to elicit something. If you are responsible for staff at work, how do they feel when they see you? What do they expect? Anchors build by repetition; if you constantly bring bad news or are always critical, you become an anchor to others for bad states. How can you be a positive anchor for them, so they feel good when you are around?

There are two ways. First, states are contagious, so when you are in a resourceful state, you are more likely to be a good anchor for others. People want to be around those who make them feel good – they may not know how it works, but they will feel it. The second way is direct. Find out what they have done right and praise them for it. Tell them exactly and specifically what they did right. Praise, like criticism, has little effect if it is too general. When you praise, you will be a pleasure to work with. If you have children, praise their behaviour specifically and remorselessly. This is the best way to build their self-esteem. We are very quick to tell children what they have done wrong, albeit with the positive intention of helping them to stop and do it right. Studies in England suggest children receive nine negatives or criticism for every positive piece of praise. For a child who wants attention, misbehaving may be the most effective way of getting it. Reinforcing the positive is just as important as discouraging the negative.

Using anchors to change state

Using anchors is the key to designing, changing and choosing your baseline state, your learning state or any other state you wish. Choose the resources you want, associate them to an anchor, and then consistently use that anchor to bring those resources into the present moment, so the state is established.

The NLP presupposition is:

We either already have all the resources we need or we can create them.

What is difficult sometimes is bringing them to where they are needed.

There are three ways to access resources.

1. *Find a role model.* You may have got your baseline state from a role model without realizing. Now you can pick one that appeals to you. When children play, they become different characters, they 'try on' different states. You can do the same. Choose a role model. It can be a real or a fictional character. 'Try on' that character for size. What would it be like to be that character? What sort of state allows them to act the way they do? What could you take from that character that is valuable for you?

2. *Use your physiology.* This is the physical approach to states. Changing your physiology is the most direct way of changing your state. A stuck state, for example, will show in stuck physiology; getting up and moving is the simplest action you can take to change state. Changing your breathing will change your state. If you are feeling anxious, slow your breathing rate and take your time to exhale. A short exhale time allows carbon dioxide to build up in the bloodstream and that produces symptoms of anxiety. It is possible to feel anxious by hyperventilating: breathing quickly and shallowly *as if* you were frightened. Smiling broadly, looking up and standing straight will change your state. Acting *as if* you feel good will start to produce those very feelings. John Grinder's work has focused on using physiology to change state and solve problems. He calls it 'Personal Editing'.

3. *Change your thinking.* One way to do this is to 'think of a time when...' For example, think of a really pleasant experience, something you want to remember and enjoy. Go back into that scene, making sure you are 'associated' in the memory – that is, seeing through

your own eyes. Hear the sounds and the voices that
are there, and enjoy the good feelings again. Come
back to the present when you are ready. You will have
changed state. The actual experience was in the past,
but this state can be a resource in the present. By
recalling an experience, you will re-experience the
state that goes with it. We do this when we reminisce
and when we look through old photograph albums
or holiday snaps or choose to play a particularly
evocative piece of music. The photographs and the
music act as anchors to help us back to those states.

It does not matter where or when you had the state you
want, you can take it to where you need it. Anchors are the
way to transfer resources from the past to the present, from
one part of our life to another. We often do not transfer
resources, thinking that they are glued to the experience that
evoked them. They are not, they are detachable.

For example, a friend of Joseph's has tremendous patience
and negotiation skills when dealing with her children. She
miraculously resolves their disputes. Yet at work, when she
was given the job of negotiating a contract on behalf of
her firm, she was very unsure of herself initially, as she did
not think she had any proper 'negotiation skills'. Then she
realized that the same principles apply as in her family:
find out what the parties want, find a point of common
agreement, trade off differences until you reach a win–win
solution and make sure you have congruent agreement from
everyone involved. She used these skills in the negotiation
and did a fine job.

Likewise Ian has a friend who has the utmost patience
when doing jigsaw puzzles yet complains he has no patience
at work when something goes wrong!

Start to notice your resource states, for it will make
them easier to access. Begin by taking a sheet of paper and

making a list of all the things that made you feel good today, however fleeting: relaxing over a cup of coffee, writing a good letter, waking refreshed, that first bite of lunch. Do this every day. Feeling good is a natural state. You do not need a logical reason for it and nobody needs to give their permission! Begin to notice positive states and collect them, like beautiful pebbles from your walk on the beach of life. Leave the old bits of wood, the sharp stones and the plastic cartons. They are there, but you do not have to tread on them or take them home.

Building a state with anchors

Here is a process that will build a resource state. First you have to decide what state you want. What resources do you want to be there? For example, you might need to face a challenge with humour, patience or curiosity.

Remember a time when you had that state and get back to it strongly – see what you saw then, hear what you heard then and get the feeling as strongly as you can. If you cannot find an example, think of a role model you can use and imagine living an episode as them where they are in the state you want. When you have identified the state you want, change state by coming back to the present.

Decide what associations or anchors you want to use to trigger that state. Pick one thing you can see in your mind's eye (a visual anchor), one sound or word you can say to yourself (an auditory anchor) and one small inconspicuous gesture you can make (a kinaesthetic anchor). Some people use a clenched fist or touching two fingers together. The picture, sound and gesture should be distinctive and memorable.

Go back and fully experience that resourceful state. See what you saw, hear what you heard and feel your full body sense. Use your physiology so your body congruently expresses that state. Just before the resourceful feeling reaches its peak, see the picture, hear the sound and make the gesture. Then change your physiology, change state and think of something else.

Test your anchors. See the picture, hear the sound and make the gesture and notice how this brings back the resourceful feeling. If you are not satisfied, go back to the resource experience again and use your anchors when you are strongly in that resource state. Then change state and test again. Do this as many times as you need, until the anchors do bring back the resourceful feeling. Anchors streamline and strengthen with use.

You have now set up your own anchors so that whenever you see that picture, hear that sound and make that gesture, it puts you into the state you want. You do not need all three anchors; indeed, some people use only one anchor. Find out what works best for you.

You can stack different states on the same anchor. To create a learning state that has curiosity, focus and commitment, go through the anchoring process for each of the three in turn, so that at the end of the process, your anchor brings up an interesting cocktail of all three. Like our friend who turned a picture upside down on his wall, you may want to set up a trigger so you remember to use the anchors. It is no use having a wonderful state cocktail at your elbow if you do not drink it.

Use this process to design a baseline state and enter it at every opportunity. You may also want to do some body work such as the Alexander Technique or Feldenkrais to change your physiology. Our bodies learn slowly and deeply, and it may take some time to change habitual unresourceful physiology.

Two final points about using anchors. They do not work by denying emotions or as emotional sticking plasters. It may be important and appropriate to feel an emotion like sadness, and using anchors to change this state will work only in the short term. Second, it is as important to be able to come out of intensely committed states as to go into them. Performing artists and athletes, for example, need to enter very intensely focused states and maintain them, and then they need a way out. The sprinter is able to make an all-out effort because there is a finishing line. When the curtain comes down, the actor must have a way of coming out of role. There are many examples of performing artists who cannot distinguish their role from their identity, and of athletes who burn out in the fast lane instead of using it only when they need to.

Our states affect us on every logical level. The ability to choose and change them is one of the most practically useful tools NLP has to offer. Once you have this, your life will be different. You will not be a victim, and you will have moved the locus of control from outside to inside yourself.

5

Reality Leaves a Lot to the Imagination

Human beings share the same five senses and the same basic neurology, yet see, hear and feel the world very differently. How do we make personal meaning from the events that befall us? First, we are not passive receivers of input, like a computer keyboard. Our brain does not sit back thinking, 'Oh, here comes a taste, here come some nice sounds.' We are active explorers of reality. Perception comes from the inside out. Every single brain is unique, and as we search out what is interesting and important to us, we strengthen certain neural connections in our brains and weaken others. We are drawn to those things that interest us. Nature does not come with labels attached. We attach them.

Our senses are the channels through which we perceive the outside world. Aldous Huxley called them the 'doors of perception' – sight, hearing, feeling, taste and smell.

Take a moment to try this simple experiment.

- Look around you. See what is in the immediate environment. Listen to any sounds and voices that are around you.

- Next pay attention to how you are feeling, your bodily sensations and any emotions you feel.

- Now pay attention to the smells, whatever they are: wood or food or car exhaust.

- Finally, what are you tasting right now?

- Here you are using your senses in the present. Now, close your eyes and think back to that experience you just had. It is a memory from a few seconds ago. Recreate it as best you can.

- Now wipe away the visual part, so there are no pictures in your mind.

- Next, delete any sounds or voices.

- Next, wipe away the feelings and the emotions. Finally delete the tastes and the smells.

- Is there anything left? If there is, delete that as well, come back to the present and open your eyes.

You recreated those experiences through your senses. There is no other way.

The NLP presupposition is:

We process all information through our senses.

Our senses are receptive to certain aspects of whatever is out there. The human eye, for example, responds to a narrow band of electromagnetic frequency which stimulates the retina and the message is passed to the visual cortex of each hemisphere for analysis. This involves connecting the new input to memories of other experiences to form a perception called 'the remembered present' by some neurologists. We project this perception back out into the world and act as if it is really out there. We are like spectators in a cinema, thinking the film is part of the screen, when it is in a spool in the projection booth. All we can say for certain is we do *not* know what is really out there.

However, being conscious, we have the ability to decide which signals from the environment are the most important at a particular time and should come into our awareness over all the possible signals. We do not throw our doors of perception wide open or we would be totally overwhelmed. We have gatekeepers that we set on the doors: beliefs, values, interests, occupations and preoccupations all patrol the threshold to preserve us from sensory overload.

Our map of reality

What we finally perceive is a map of reality. Some parts are full of detail, others are sketchy and some may be completely empty. Having made our map, is it a good one? Is it well signposted and does it make it easy or difficult to get what we want?

One of the most important NLP presuppositions is:

People respond to their map of reality and not to reality itself.

'The map is not the territory', in the phrase coined by Alfred Korzybski in his book *Science and Sanity*, published in 1933. NLP is the art of changing our map for one that gives us more choice. It works like the wise man in the story of the 17 camels.

A man died, leaving his entire estate to be divided between his three sons. The eldest was to have one half, the second to have one third and the youngest to have one ninth of the total. The only problem was that the estate consisted of 17 camels. The sons were on the verge of killing a camel and cutting it up, when the wise man came riding into the story on his camel.

On hearing the dilemma he said to the three sons, 'Here, take my camel as a gift. Add it to yours so you have 18. Now, you, the oldest son, get half, that is nine camels. The middle son gets a third – six camels. The youngest gets a ninth, that is two camels. Correct?'

The sons are satisfied.

'That is a total of 17 camels,' said the wise man. 'By a happy chance my camel is left over.'

He mounts his camel and rides away.

Representational systems

You make your map and you have to live in it. Remember two things as you create it:

1. How you use your senses on the *outside* is going to affect your thinking and experience on the *inside.*

2. You can change your experience by changing how you use your senses on the inside.

We have an incredible ability to create experience on the inside. Our brain is a natural virtual reality machine. Who needs a special helmet? A painful memory will make us wince again. A pleasant memory will make us smile and re-experience the pleasure. Imagine eating a lemon and you will salivate. We represent our experience to ourselves using our senses, so in NLP the senses are called *representational systems.* There are five representational systems:

- sight (visual, abbreviated to V)

- hearing (auditory, abbreviated to A)

- feeling (kinaesthetic, abbreviated to K)

- tasting (gustatory, abbreviated to G)

- smell (olfactory, abbreviated to O).

There are some distinctions within the systems. Many people use the auditory system to talk to themselves, and for some people, this is what 'thinking' is. It *is* one way of thinking, but not the only way. The kinaesthetic system is made up of feelings of balance (the vestibular system), bodily feelings from within and direct tactile feelings of touch from outside.

There are also our emotions, feelings *about* some person or situation. These are clusters of feelings in our body and we label them: for example, fright, anxiety, love and hate.

From moment to moment we create our internal world using our representational systems. We are experts; we can create some wonderful sensory cocktails. Once you know you create your internal world, you can start to create it the way you want it, rather than the way your brain does by default. Just as we develop skill and preferences in using our senses on the outside, so we do the same with our representational systems on the inside. What are your preferences? With a visual preference you may be interested in drawing, interior design and fashion, the visual arts, television, films, art therapy and symbolism, painting, mathematics and physics. With an auditory preference you may be interested in language, writing, drama, music, talking approaches to therapy, training and lecturing. A kinaesthetic preference might be manifested in sport, carpentry, gymnastics, body work therapies and athletics. The more you use your senses on the outside and the more acute they are, the more you may favour them as representational systems. This does not mean you are typecast, only that you have certain strengths – and perhaps certain weaknesses if you tend *not* to use a particular representational system.

Know your preferences. Know your strengths and potentials. Many people think they have no talent for music, art or mathematics, when in fact they are just not using the best representational system for the task. Music involves the ability to hear internal sounds, while art and design need the visual system. Academic learning, particularly in the sciences, needs the ability to access a lot of information at once, and to do this you need to use the visual system. Children who do not use the visual system usually find formal school education difficult, so they need to be taught to visualize. One fact we have both found in our work is that when we teach people to develop their representational systems, they become naturally talented in ways they had not been before.

When you recreate an experience, you are likely to use one of the systems to open up the experience for you. This is known as the *lead system*. If it is the visual system it will act like an icon on a computer – you click on it and the whole program will open. An auditory lead system is like hearing the first few notes of a piece of music and immediately knowing what it is. A kinaesthetic lead gives you the feeling that suddenly transports you back to the complete memory.

Learning styles

Representational systems link with different learning styles. Theories of learning all agree that for maximum impact learners need to see what they are learning – visual displays, graphs and diagrams. They need to hear what they are learning – lectures, talks, tapes and music – and they need to experience it – role plays, practice and rehearsal. When education is a multi-sensory experience, not only is it more interesting and more fun, but it also caters for every preference by using all the representational systems. So-called 'slow' learners are often just 'different' learners; they find the current teaching style hard to relate to. University education in particular often concentrates on lectures, tuning in to the auditory learners, but not giving sufficient attention to those students who favour the visual and kinaesthetic representational systems. The danger for teachers and presenters is that they may give the perfect presentation in just the way they themselves would find it easiest to learn the material and ignore other systems.

Relationships

Representational systems are very important too in understanding your relationships. First, how do we know someone cares about us? For some people this is mostly visual. They need to see demonstrations of affection and loving looks. Giving and receiving gifts may be important, and they will take care of their appearance and expect others to do the same. When their partner looks good this is evidence that he or she cares about them.

Others need to hear continually how much the other person cares. A loving tone of voice is very important, and they will be particularly sensitive to the words and tone that others use. They may be less forgiving of words spoken in anger or jest, because for them, words are important. They like to talk and discuss issues with those they care about. They may use their voice tone to express how they feel and expect others to hear the message.

There are others who are more kinaesthetic and want physical demonstrations of affection. Without them, they may believe the other person has ceased to care and feel rejected.

Couples need to know what is important to each other. One partner may feel unloved because the other is not demonstrating affection in the way that they recognize. For example, if the auditory channel is important, they want to hear their partner tell them that they love them. They may be blind to loving glances. This is fertile ground for arguments and misunderstandings.

We also tend to choose as our friends people with the same dominant representational system, because we will have many interests in common.

When you know how people think, you can understand what is important to them and also what really annoys them. People who favour the visual system are likely to be put off by a messy or untidy environment. Perhaps you have a work colleague whose desk is always neat and who always knows where things are? They are likely to be visual. People who are predominantly auditory may be easily disturbed by noise. They need a quiet place to work. Others who are more kinaesthetic like to be comfortable; they are sensitive to how and where they are sitting. As long as they are comfortable, they may be able to work in a noisy, untidy environment that will drive their colleagues crazy. When you know about representational systems, you can understand how people can be so different. You can both arrange your own work conditions in the way that suits you best and understand and respect the needs of others.

The physiology of thinking

How we think shows in our physiology. Here is the NLP presupposition that has been implicit in much of what we have discussed:

The mind and body are one system.

Think about cartoons for a moment. Cartoons are costly and time consuming, and so animators want to convey information about the character as economically as possible. There is no running commentary that tells you when or how the character is thinking and feeling, so certain gestures are used consistently to convey certain emotions, states and experiences, because they are presumed to be immediately understandable (see Figure 5.1).

What is the physiology that goes with visualizing? People who are visualizing will tend to be looking up or level and their neck muscles are likely to be contracted. They may also furrow their brow as if trying to focus on something (they are). People who spend a lot of time visualizing may complain of headaches or a stiff neck. It is possible, however, to see clear mental pictures while relaxing the neck muscles.

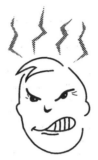

Figure 5.1 Anger

Breathing is a critical part of physiology. When visualizing, people tend to stand or sit erect and breathe high in the chest. Breathing like this results in shorter, more shallow breaths, so people who are visualizing will tend to breathe and speak more quickly.

The physiology that goes with auditory thinking is different. Here there may be small rhythmic movements of the body, often swaying from side to side. The voice tonality will be clear, expressive, often musical. Do you know anyone who habitually puts their head on one side when they think? Some people will lean their head on their hand as if speaking on the telephone. This is called the 'telephone position'. They are listening to voices and sounds inside their head. You may also see their lips move as they form the words they are saying to themselves.

Kinaesthetic thinking is thinking with the body and will usually involve a rounded, even slumped posture. When people think this way, they will often look downwards, for this helps to get in touch with bodily feelings. They will tend to breathe abdominally, low in the body, and the voice is often lower and slower, because abdominal breathing is fuller and slower. Feelings are slower to manifest than pictures, so a conversation between someone who is thinking visually and someone who is thinking kinaesthetically can be frustrating for both sides. The visual thinker may become impatient because the kinaesthetic thinker speaks more slowly and takes longer to reply. The kinaesthetic thinker may feel hurried and become uncomfortable.

We do not suggest that there is such a thing as a universal body language. We all use all the representational systems and very many people will habitually favour one system. This being so, their physiology may take on some of these characteristics, just as our features are moulded over time by our habitual expressions into laugh lines, furrowed brows or pursed lips. Physiology is summarized in Table 5.1.

TABLE 5.1 REPRESENTATIONAL SYSTEM PHYSIOLOGY

	Visual	Auditory	Kinaesthetic
Posture	head up erect	often swaying, head tilted to one side, 'telephone position'	rounded, head down
Breathing	high in chest	mid-range	low in abdomen
Voice and tonality	fast, voice higher pitched	melodic, rhythmic	lower and softer
Eye movements	up or defocus	midline or down left	down or down right

Eye accessing cues

Watch eye movements. Have you ever wondered what they mean? You may have noticed that there is some pattern and purpose to them. Eyes do not flop around randomly inside their sockets, subject to gravity when we lean over. NLP suggests that there is a link between the way our eyes move and the way we think.

Eye movements are known as *eye accessing cues* in NLP literature, because they enable us to access certain information. They cue us. Figure 5.2 illustrates this.

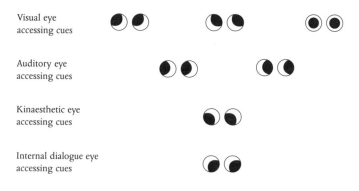

Visual eye
accessing cues

Auditory eye
accessing cues

Kinaesthetic eye
accessing cues

Internal dialogue eye
accessing cues

Figure 5.2 Eye accessing cues
(Note: This is as you look at another person)

There seems to be an innate connection between eye movements and representational systems. Particular eye movements are linked to particular systems. In general, people will look upwards or defocus when they visualize. They will move their eyes sideways to the left or right when hearing sounds internally and they may look down to their right when thinking kinaesthetically. Looking down to their left usually signifies internal dialogue. These movements are consistent and mostly unconscious. They are the general patterns, so do not take these as true for everyone all of the time.

It is possible to start exploring eye movements in ordinary conversation. Sit down with a friend and ask them some questions. Pay attention to their eye movements, not their answers. Start with questions or instructions where they need to visualize; for example:

'Visualize your front door.'

'Imagine what I would look like with green hair.'

'Which one of your friends is the tallest?'

Examples of auditory questions and instructions would be:

'Listen to some of your favourite music in your mind.'

'How many words are there in the first verse of the national anthem?'

'What would your voice sound like under water?'

For internal dialogue, simply ask them to have an engrossing conversation with themselves about some topic that interests them.

For feelings, ask them what it is like to step into a hot bath or which hand is warmer.

What are the practical applications of eye accessing cues? You can use them not only to find out how others are thinking but also to make it easier for yourself to think in particular ways: you are literally tuning into your body and mind, like tuning into a television programme. When you need to visualize, look up. When you need to contact your feelings, look down. Use accessing cues to help you think more precisely and clearly in the way you want to.

When you are teaching or training you can also use eye accessing cues. For example, if you use visual aids such as a flip chart, position them ideally up and to the left of the viewers. This makes it easier for them to access the visual memory.

Accessing cues are a metaphor for how we use our brain. Some parts of our brains are familiar and some accessing cues come easily. Other parts may be uncharted country and we may not use those accessing cues much, if at all. People who have had traumatic experiences may block off certain channels so as not to bring up painful memories. Are there places you do not go to very often in, say, your visual field? Well, how can you have clear *visions* of the future unless you *look* in the right place? Use accessing cues to claim all the parts of your brain. This could be the single most important thing you could experiment with to improve your creativity and range of thought.

Eye accessing cues have another practical use in pacing or helping others. Joseph once worked with a professional violinist. She had a regular job playing with an orchestra in one of the London theatres. She complained of being nervous and distracted when she played, assailed by a self-doubting internal dialogue. She shared a music stand with another violinist, who stood on her left. The music stand was between them, so she was always looking down to her left to read the music. Looking down to the left will often access internal dialogue. She changed the position of the music and the internal dialogue disappeared. Simple and effective.

People who become depressed will habitually look down to their right. When they say they cannot see any future, they are absolutely right, for they are looking in the wrong place. A colleague of ours was working with a badly depressed person. As he persuaded her to look up more and more, she started to see more possibilities, a brighter future for her life. But after a while, she would slip back into looking down and these possibilities seemed to disappear. He said to her, 'When you are sitting and looking up here, you seem to see some possibilities and ways forward. Yes?' She agreed. 'Why don't you keep looking up there?' She said that it was unfamiliar. It was as if she had to learn a different physiology. He persevered, and the work they did together marked the beginning of the end of her habitual depression. This is not to suggest an instant cure for depression. For us, the lesson is how habitual our way of being can become. Habitual body posture links with habitual thoughts. And even if our particular way of organizing our physiology is positively life-threatening, it still affords us the comfort of familiarity. Our postures and thoughts can become so familiar that in the end they seem to be the way things are. In fact they are our own creations.

Speaking your mind

Language is rich and flexible and there are many different ways to express our thoughts. You have probably had the experience of searching for just the right word to express yourself and some come to mind, but they will not do. People will also express the same idea differently using language from different representational systems. For example, we have friends who say, 'Be seeing you.' Some say, 'I'll be hearing from you.' Others will say, 'I'll be in contact.'

NLP understands language as a reflection of inner experience. It is a surprisingly accurate translation of the way we think. Our words speak volumes once we have an ear for sensory language. For example, our last sentence was full of words about the sense of hearing. The words and phrases that show which internal sense we are using are called *predicates* and *predicate phrases* in NLP.

Imagine three people describing a house. The first says, 'The house is a magnificent *sight*. The main room is huge and *looks* out onto the garden and there is a great *view* across the park. The *colour* scheme is beautifully co-ordinated and we were *shown* round everything. It's *clear* we will buy it. I *foresee* a very happy time living there.'

The second says, 'We quite liked the house. The estate agent *told* us a lot about its history. I thought the decorations were a bit *loud* and the garden is nothing to *shout* about. The *noise* of the railway track was a bit intrusive. We did not really feel in *tune* with the neighbourhood. I'll have to *talk* it over further before deciding.'

The third person says, 'I got a strong *feeling* that we would not be happy here. It just isn't a place I could feel *comfortable* living in. I can't really put my *finger* on anything *concrete*. I don't want to be *pushed* into a decision now and I do not want to *hold* anyone up. I will *contact* the estate agent tomorrow.'

They are talking about the same house, each noticing different things and thinking about it in different ways. The first was visual, the second auditory and the third kinaesthetic.

Here are other common predicates to show you how they sound, so you can get a feel for the idea:

Visual words and phrases

Look, focus, imagination, see, watch, colour, dim, notice, illustrate, reveal, insight, blank, perspective.

I see what you mean.
Something to look forward to.
It colours his view of life.
A dark cloud on the horizon.
The future looks bright.
Taking a dim view.
My point of view.

Auditory words and phrases

Say, loud, sound, deaf, remark, discuss, speechless, silence, listen, music, harmony.

On the same wavelength.
Turn a deaf ear.
Speak your mind.
Word for word.
Loud and clear.
What do you say?

Kinaesthetic words and phrases (including taste and smell)

Touch, solid, warm, cold, rough, grasp, hold, gentle, heavy, weak, hot, smooth, move.

Get to grips with the idea.
Hold on a moment.
A cool customer.
Put your finger on it.
Heated argument.
A smooth operator.

Olfactory words and phrases

Nose, smell, pungent, fragrant.

Smell a rat.
Smelling of roses.
A nose for business.

Gustatory words and phrases

Spicy, sweet, bitter, salty.

A bitter experience.
A taste for the good life.
Saccharine sweet.

There are also unspecified words that do not belong to any one representation system: idea, decide, think, know, learn, change, operate, meditate, understand.

Know yourself and pace others

Sensory-based language is a powerful tool in communicating and influencing.

First, know yourself. Find out your own language and thinking preferences. You can do this by writing or speaking into a tape recorder for a few minutes about your personal and professional life. Don't think about it, just write or say whatever comes into your head. Then notice what language predominates – seeing, hearing or feeling.

Start to notice how others express their thoughts. This is rather like learning a foreign language. Listen in the moment to what sensory-based words people use and over time you will probably start to hear patterns. A person will consistently use language from their preferred representational system, so listening to them is the easiest way to find out which one they favour. Listen past the content of what a person says to how he says it. This is fascinating – a whole series of multi-sensory worlds will open up in front of you. Like eye movements, they were always there. You have opened the doors of perception a fraction more.

Once you have developed an ear for sensory language you will be able to pace others with language. Use words from the same representation system as they do. This will give you rapport on the verbal level. For example, someone says, 'I can't *tell* if this is right for me.' You reply, 'What more do you need to *hear*?' If they were to talk instead about getting a clear *vision* and then moving forward, you would pace them by talking in terms of *seeing* the way forward.

Ian was called in as a consultant to a manufacturing company because two directors were arguing about policy. Both had excellent qualities and were not using them fully because of the conflict. It only took one meeting to resolve the problem. The first director, James, thought Fred was out of touch and unsympathetic. Fred thought James was short-sighted and a fuzzy thinker. James was more kinaesthetic, Fred more visual. Fred slowed down his rate of talking, which helped rapport between them. Ian took Fred's vision of the company and translated it into kinaesthetic words for James, something he could relate to. At the end of the meeting, both directors were basically in agreement. James would deal with the public relations side and Fred would focus on overall planning. Before they had difficulty communicating because they had been speaking different languages. They needed a translator!

In teaching, training or writing, use a mixture of hearing, seeing and feeling words. Become adept at clothing your thoughts in the different types of predicate. Let the visual people see what you mean, the auditory thinkers hear you loud and clear and the feeling thinkers get a grasp of your main points. The more vivid your language, the more vivid the experience for the learner.

The same principles apply to your writing. The hardest prose to read is technical papers full of abstract words with no sight or sound of relief. Abstract subjects do not have to be explained in abstract language.

Thought connects with physiology and both connect with language. The next chapter will further explore how our maps of reality are translated into the skills we have and words we speak.

6

Customizing
Your Brain

Submodalities

The five representational systems – seeing, feeling, hearing, tasting and smelling – are the building blocks of our internal experience and are sometimes known as *modalities*.

Any distinction we can make with our senses in the outside world, we can also make in our inner world. For example, we see colours and sense distance in our mental world as well as in the outside world. In NLP these distinctions are called *submodalities*. Submodalities are the smaller building blocks of the senses, the way complete pictures, sounds and feelings are composed. They are the qualities that make each experience distinct.

Make yourself comfortable and remember a pleasant memory. Look at your mental picture of it. If you find it hard to visualize, see whatever you can. Is the picture black and white or is it in colour? Is it moving or still? How bright is it? Are you looking at the scene through your own eyes or are you seeing yourself in the picture? These are all examples of visual submodalities. Let the picture fade.

Now listen to any sounds and voices in your memory. Are they loud or soft, near or far? Are they continuous? Are they clear or muffled? From which direction do they come? These are auditory submodalities. Let the sounds fade.

Now the feelings. Whereabouts in your body are they located? Is each feeling large or small? Warm or cool? How intense is it? How large is the area it covers? These are kinaesthetic submodalities. Let these feelings fade.

Our memories, hopes and beliefs all have a submodality structure, and this is how we give them meaning. Then we have feelings *about* them. This is true whether they are unique events, for example 'my first date', or classes of experience, for example 'love', 'beliefs', 'confusion' or 'hobbies'.

Here are some of the most common submodality distinctions. There may also be others that are important to you.

Visual submodalities

- associated (seen through own eyes) or dissociated (looking on at self)

- colour or black and white

- framed or unbounded

- depth (two- or three-dimensional)

- location (e.g. to left or right, up or down)

- distance of self from picture

- brightness

- contrast

- clarity (blurred or focused)

- movement (like a film or a slide show)

- speed (faster or slower than usual)

- number (split screen or multiple images)

- size

Auditory submodalities

- stereo or mono
- words or sounds
- volume (loud or soft)
- tone (soft or harsh)
- timbre (fullness of sound)
- location of sound
- distance from sound source
- duration
- continuous or discontinuous
- speed (faster or slower than usual)
- clarity (clear or muffled)

Kinaesthetic submodalities

- location
- intensity
- pressure (hard or soft)
- extent (how big)
- texture (rough or smooth)
- weight (light or heavy)
- temperature
- duration (how long it lasts)
- shape

Using submodalities

Submodalities offer tremendous opportunities for gaining control of our subjective experience because we can change them at any time. Take, for example, your experience of a negative state, say boredom. How is it possible to experience boredom? Whatever the outside cause, the state itself will have a submodality structure. For example, when people describe being bored, they will typically talk about everything being 'flat' or 'grey'. They will use a typical tone of voice.

To change a state of boredom, determine its submodality structure in all representational systems. Then think of a state you would rather be in, for example curiosity. Think of something you are very curious about and again determine the submodality structure of that state. Now take a step back and look at both sets of submodalities. How are they different? Go back to the bored experience (if you still can) and change the submodalities of boredom to those of curiosity. Notice how your experience is different.

When you are in a bored state, you cannot 'make' yourself curious by will-power, however much you may want to be. But changing submodalities gives you the practical means to change your state.

> When we change the structure of the experience by changing the submodalities, then the meaning will also change. When the meaning changes, our internal response will also change.

Some submodality changes will have a particularly powerful effect on your internal experience. These are known as *critical submodalities.*

As language both reflects and triggers inner experience, submodalities form the basis of predicate phrases, those sensory sayings and metaphors in everyday speech. Submodality phrases are often true and literal representations, and so can actually evoke and change the submodalities of the way experiences are represented. For example, we are focusing in on these ideas, turning them over and looking at them from different angles. Think about opening up a subject – how does it feel different from closing it down? Once you have closed it down, slammed the lid shut, put the subject on the back burner or out in the cold, it becomes very difficult to think about. Once you open up an idea, you can expand it, frame it and smooth out any problems. Although becoming skilful with this type of conversational submodality change may seem a far cry, when the subject attracts you, mastery is not far off.

Understanding submodalities gives you a way of having more choices about your experience. They are an essential part of the badly needed and yet unwritten 'Brain User's Manual'. Let's now look at how submodality metaphors reflect our experience of time.

Timelines

We talk about time using a rich mixture of submodality expressions. We use them to code our subjective experience of it. Without some way of sorting time, we would be in serious trouble.

Whatever time really is, our subjective experience of it seems to be spatial. We use metaphors like 'looking forward to holidays', 'going back in time', 'a long way in the past', 'the distant future'. We seem to think of time as a line. Have you ever thought about how we distinguish the past, present and future? When you think about an event in the past, how do you know when (or even if) it happened? How do you know something happened two weeks ago and not two months or two years ago?

Where would you locate your past? Think of a past event. Where is it? Point in that direction. Now, where would you locate your future? Think of something you hope to be doing soon and point in that direction. Imagine a line that connects your past with your future. That is your *timeline*. To find out another person's timeline, ask them to compare an event that happened in the past with one they hope for in the future. Listen to how they talk about each event, and particularly watch which way they look and gesture. Their body knows where their past and future are, even if they are not consciously aware of it.

Timelines tend to fall into two categories. The first is called *in time*. People who are in time usually have their timeline running from front to back – the past is literally behind them, the future in front. They live in the 'now' part of the timeline, so are not usually aware of the passage of time and are more spontaneous and may find it difficult to be punctual and meet deadlines. These are the people who open their diary for the forthcoming week and are horrified to see how much is in it. It is as if it takes them by surprise.

The second category is *through time*. The through time person has the past, present and future all in front of them. Usually the past runs to the left and the future to the right. Through time people are good planners. They will be punctual and are good at time management.

Figure 6.1 illustrates both in time and through time.

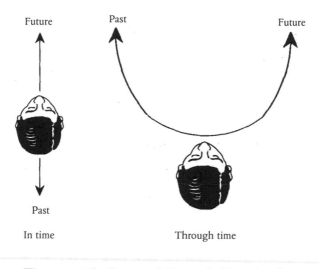

Figure 6.1 In time and through time timelines

Timelines have fascinating implications. Some people are poor time managers and this can be important in business – Western business culture is typically through time. One lady we know had a well-deserved reputation for being late for meetings. When we asked her where she kept her past memories and future plans, she gestured vaguely in front of her on the floor. 'They are all in there together,' she said. This lady also sometimes thinks she has done something when she in fact has not. Knowing how she stores time, this is hardly surprising.

It is important to pace a person's way of organizing time. Then they may be motivated to adjust their timeline in a way that would help them be more effective. Time management courses are by through time people for through time people. The people they are designed to help, the in time people, find them difficult to use!

We use timelines in NLP in a variety of ways – gaining access to memories in the past, in therapy and time management, and for creating compelling futures. There is a wide and fascinating NLP literature on timelines.

Associated and dissociated states

Association and dissociation are two very important submodalities. You are associated when you are inside an experience, seeing it through your own eyes. You are dissociated from an experience when you are outside it, seeing yourself at one remove.

Think of a pleasant experience, one you would like to relive now. As you remember it, are you associated or dissociated, or do you seem to flicker between the two states?

Now change state. Move your body and think back to a mildly unpleasant experience and relive it now. Are you associated, dissociated or going between the two states? Change state again.

An associated experience is very different from a dissociated experience. When you are associated, you are in the experience and you get the bodily feelings, good or bad, 'associated' with the experience. Store pleasant memories as associated pictures to enjoy them again. When you are dissociated, you are outside the experience and do not experience the accompanying feelings. You might have wondered how it is possible for some people to look back on important and intense experiences and say they feel nothing. They do it by dissociating.

Dissociating can be very useful; it keeps the feelings from painful memories at bay. It also enables you to learn from the experience. Think for a moment of a negative experience in the past. Notice whether you are associated or dissociated as you recall it. If you are associated, then dissociate. Step out of yourself, leave your body in the picture and see yourself in the scene. If you are already dissociated, then change your perspective, look at yourself from a different angle, perhaps from above or below, or retreat even further away. Now, as you see yourself in that situation, what can you learn from it?

You have used submodalities to change the way you experience in order to learn something you might otherwise have missed.

These associated and dissociated perspectives are more than just states of mind. They register in your body. When you are associated, you are in the present moment, aware of your body and your feelings. An associated state is *in time.* You may be leaning forward. You have probably seen other people leaning forward, being drawn into an intense argument or discussion. You can see they are associating and you know for yourself what this is like.

When you are dissociated, you feel slightly distant, 'not quite with it', in a reflective mood. You are objective and thinking *about* things, planning the future or contemplating the past. A dissociated state is *through time.* Your body is likely to be 'laid back'.

Neither association nor dissociation is better. Both are useful; it depends what you want to do. Some activities you will definitely want to be associated into, some you will want to dissociate from. To be able to move freely between each gives you a great deal of emotional freedom and scope for learning. Sometimes people are stuck in one mode, often the dissociated if they have suffered a great deal in the past.

Our body awareness also has a submodality structure, and so do self-esteem and physical health. The way we think of ourselves affects our body, for mind and body are connected. These images and feelings are often unconscious. A great deal of work has been done in mind–body medicine on the power of visualization in health and illness. Visualization is more powerful if patients are taught how to give their images the submodalities of health. Our internal dialogue, or self talk, also affects our health. An internal dialogue that is constantly telling you how bad you feel wears you down. NLP suggests your immune system is eavesdropping on your internal dialogue.

Modelling

In NLP, *modelling* means finding out how someone does something. It is the core of NLP, the process of replicating excellence. Modelling a skill means finding out how the person who has the skill thinks about it, and the beliefs and values that enable them to do it. You can also model emotions, experiences, behaviour, beliefs and values. NLP models what is possible. It is possible because human beings have already done it.

The NLP presupposition is:

Modelling successful performance leads to excellence. If one person can do something it is possible to model it and teach it to others.

Modelling is a child's primary way of learning. It is how we learnt to walk and talk. Indeed, Mark Twain remarked that if we had been formally taught these skills, we would all stutter and stumble. Children simply copy the adults around them who already do what the children want to learn. So, not only do looks run in families, but also expressions, postures, voice tones, ways of reacting, attitudes, beliefs and values – and all the benefits and disadvantages these carry with them.

Although informal, modelling is powerful – skills acquired this way last longer than knowledge learnt at school.

To model a skill you focus on three neurological levels: what the model does (their behaviour and physiology), how they do it (the way they think) and why they do it (beliefs and values). You will also need to take into account the environment and the identity of the model.

To model a skill you need:

- the model's behaviour and physiology
- the way they think
- their beliefs and values.

NLP modelling has three main phases. The first phase is observing, questioning and being with the model when they are actually engaged in the skill you are interested in. You take second position with the model, becoming them as far as you are able. Direct questioning on its own can be disappointing, for a person who is very skilful has usually forgotten the learning stages and is unaware of exactly how they do the task. This is why the best performers do not necessarily make the best teachers. The work of the NLP modeller is to go beyond this barrier of consciousness and learn about the unconscious competence of the model. It is rather like trying to imagine how a complex building was constructed once the scaffolding has gone.

When you have finished the first phase you will have a lot of information, and you will not yet be sure what is important and what is not. Some elements may be the personal style of the model. So the second phase is systematically to take out each facet of the model's behaviour to find out whether it makes a difference to the results you get. If it does, then it is an essential part of the model. If it does not, then it can be relinquished.

The third and final phase is to analyse what you have learned so that you can teach it to others.

Modelling is very pragmatic and driven by results. Models cannot be right or wrong, they either work or not. This is why NLP is so strong on practical applications, for its techniques are modelled on real achievements.

There is an alternative way of modelling, which works better for some skills. Here you break the task down into small pieces and systematically set about acquiring them one by one until you have built the whole skill. This can work well, although there is a danger of finishing with a Frankenstein model patched together instead of an organic whole. Whichever way you do it, you are only finished when you can get roughly the same results as the model. Then you know it works.

NLP has generated many models, some of very complex skills: leadership, communication and language patterns, the skills of top salespeople, managers and athletes. NLP has also modelled speed-reading, spelling and musical memory. Once you have the skills of modelling, you can use them to model whatever interests you.

Mental strategies

Finding out how a person thinks – their mental strategies – is an important part of modelling. Mental strategies are how you organize your thoughts and actions to accomplish a task – from something simple, such as remembering a name, to something very complex, such as planning a career or falling in love. Just as large goals decompose into smaller tasks, complex strategies contain a number of smaller ones like a series of Chinese boxes one inside another.

To model a strategy you need to discover:

- the representation systems used

- the submodalities of the inner pictures, sounds and feelings

- the sequence of steps.

Sales strategy

Ian worked with a car company, modelling some of their best salespeople. They would invariably show the customer the car first, walking round it and admiring the bodywork. Then they would adjust the seat for the customer so that they were completely comfortable and then go for a test drive. During the drive they would remain silent. When they came back to the showroom, they would look round the car again with the customer, perhaps showing them what was under the bonnet (which was visually impressive) and only then start to talk about the car afterwards in the office. This is a selling strategy that starts with visual, then goes to kinaesthetic, returns to visual and then goes to auditory. One member of that sales team had less success than the others. He talked continually when the customer was driving, telling them about the gadgets and the features, so the customer could not concentrate on the driving. Having isolated the key elements, Ian was able to coach this salesperson quite specifically on how to improve his performance – let the car speak for itself!

Spelling strategy

The NLP spelling strategy is a good example of how important it is to use the right representational system. Writing is a visual representation of language, so a spelling strategy must involve the visual system. Good spellers of English nearly always go through the same strategy: they visualize the word as they spell it and then check if it feels right.

People who spell poorly usually do it from the sound. Unlike Italian, English words do not follow simple rules where the sound corresponds to the spelling. Good spellers can usually spell words backwards as well as forwards and, if you have the opportunity to watch them, you will see them looking up or defocusing as they visualize.

Submodalities will be important. Joseph worked with a girl who was having difficulty with spelling at school. She was visualizing the words. She looked up, but then said she could not see them very well. He asked her what colour the letters were. 'Black,' she said. He then asked her what colour the background was. 'Black,' she replied. No wonder she could not see them very well! Joseph suggested that a white background would make the letters easier to see. His pupil changed the background to white and her spelling improved so much that in a fortnight she had moved to the top spelling group in her class.

Modelling and strategies are the road to accelerated learning. With an effective learning strategy children learn quickly, naturally and easily. Teaching good learning strategies will improve the results of all students. 'Talent' at a particular subject is the result of having a good learning strategy. NLP is the basis of an education system wherein we could all learn to be naturally talented.

Motivation strategies

Have you ever wondered how you motivate yourself to do something? Your motivation strategy will determine how easily you can get down and do a task. For example, one person we modelled looks first at the work she needs to do and hears a loud, encouraging, internal voice saying, 'Time to do this.' Then she constructs a big, bright, shiny, mental picture of the finished work. Feeling good as she looks at that picture, she starts the work. This strategy works well and is pleasant to run. It moves towards a positive purpose.

Compare this with another person we modelled who looks at the work to be done and hears a nagging, nasal internal voice saying, 'Hey, you really *should* get on with this.' He feels resistant, and no wonder. He makes bright pictures of everything else he *could* do and feels better. Then he makes a picture of the consequences of not doing the work and feels bad. Not surprisingly, he goes with the pictures that make him feel good and leaves the task. He does this until the consequences of not doing the work loom so large and close and the feeling becomes so bad that he does the task. This strategy is not pleasant to run. It is fuelled by avoiding the negative consequences. Our second subject has a strategy with all four of the elements that make motivation very difficult:

1. He imagines the negative consequences of not doing the task and so associates bad feeling with the work.

2. He does not pace himself, but bullies himself in an authoritarian way.

3. He looks at the task *all at once* rather than at the steps and stages, so it looks daunting.

4. He imagines himself doing it rather than having done it.

If you want a procrastination strategy, this is one of the best. It works perfectly – if you want to always be under the pressure of deadlines.

This brings us to another NLP presupposition:

People work perfectly.

No one is wrong or broken. It is a matter of finding out how they function so that this can effectively be changed to something giving more useful or desirable results.

Anxiety strategies

As we have just seen, strategies create results, either pleasant or unpleasant. A strategy for feeling anxious is to create a series of big, bright, close pictures of all the possible things that could go wrong. Looking at these pictures will make you feel bad.

When you are anxious about someone who has stayed out late, for example, you may experience a lot of bad feelings while vividly imagining everything that might have happened to them. Then you get angry with them, holding them responsible for the feelings. They may not be very considerate, but *you* have created the pictures and the feelings, not them. Remember, we have wonderful creative mental powers and we can choose the feelings we create in ourselves.

Strategy for learning and generating choice

We would like to finish this section by giving a strategy for generating new choices in a difficult situation:

1. Think of an unsatisfactory situation in the past, one in which you would want to react differently in future. See yourself in your mind's eye at the beginning of the incident as though you were watching it on a video. Pause your mental video a fraction before the situation went downhill.

2. Ask yourself, 'What would be more effective here in creating the result that I intended?' Watch yourself doing this alternative behaviour on your mental video, instead of what actually happened. Stay dissociated while you check this alternative.

3. Now step into your 'movie', so you are associated. Be back in this situation and act in the new way that you have decided would be better. Experience it as fully as you can, seeing, hearing and feeling everything that happens. Enjoy acting out what might have been. As you act it out, again check that it works well. If it does not feel right, come out, think of another alternative, watch yourself doing it and go through the process again until you are completely satisfied both from the viewpoint of watching yourself and the viewpoint of actually doing it.

4. Finally ask yourself, 'What will let me know that it is time to use this new behaviour?' and identify exactly what you would see, hear or feel, internally or externally, that would act as your automatic cue to use this new behaviour. Next time a similar situation comes up, you will be ready for it – the new choice will be mentally rehearsed and available.

This is a general strategy that can be used to learn from what has happened and come up with specific new actions that would work better.

7

The Gatekeepers at the Doors of Perception

How do we create our model of the world from our experience? There are three gatekeepers at the doors of perception.

1. *Deletion.* We are selective about our experience and leave parts out – we delete them. Either they do not register or we discount them as unimportant. If you have ever searched for your keys and found them in a place you had already looked, you will know how deletion works.

2. *Distortion.* We change our experience, amplifying or diminishing it, and seeing it differently, as if in a fairground hall of mirrors.

3. *Generalization.* We take certain aspects of our experience as representative of a whole class and pay no attention to exceptions. This is useful because it lets us respond to new situations on the basis of what we have learned from similar ones in the past. It is a problem if we generalize wrongly or do not stay open to new experience. Beliefs are examples of generalizations.

These gatekeepers are neither good nor bad in themselves; they are both an asset and a liability. If we did not delete some sensory information we would be overwhelmed.

However, we may be deleting just what we need to pay attention to, for example how we are feeling or important feedback from others. Sometimes we hear the negative in what others say and delete the positive, even when they are both in the same sentence.

In the same way, if we did not distort we would stifle our creativity. When you are planning to redecorate, it is useful to be able to imagine what a room is going to look like when it is finished. This is sensory distortion. But if you decide that when someone looks at you in a certain way they are really despising you, you run the risk of distorting the meaning of their look and then distorting your response. Fantasy builds on fantasy.

When you generalize you aim to make sense of the world and know what to expect. This means that when you encounter a door handle that is differently shaped from any you have seen before, you do not have to retire puzzled. You know that it is just another kind of handle. So generalization is a basic part of how we learn. But the same process can spell disaster. Suppose you had a difficult relationship and decided on the basis of that experience that all men or all women are the same – not to be trusted. Your generalization could stop you seeking out men and women who are exceptions to your rule.

So, through deleting, distorting and generalizing, we can create a friendly or a hostile world. And the more we practise, the better we will get at making the world fit our filters.

People have biases on how they shape their perceptions. Some people will do more deleting, while others tend to distort more and yet others will be more given to generalization. What does this mean in practice?

People who delete a great deal make big leaps in their thinking and may be difficult to follow. They are also likely to have good powers of concentration, being able to delete distractions, and they may be good at tolerating physical discomfort.

People who distort their experience constantly surprise you with their interpretations of your actions and words. They may see cause and effect links where you would never suspect them. They make unusual connections and are likely to try to deduce your thoughts and feelings from what you say. They may also be very creative. Art, music and literature all use distortions. Distortion can create the worlds of Hieronymus Bosch or David Hockney, Stephen King or Charles Dickens.

People who generalize a lot may be very sure of themselves (or very unsure). The world may seem very simple to them. They live in a black and white world – shades of grey are not so easy to accommodate if experience has to be one thing or the other. They may also have a lot of rules of conduct to cover different situations. Scientific laws are generalizations, and the scientific method is a good way to operate: experiment, generalize from the results, but always be prepared to revise in the face of exceptions to the rule.

These last three paragraphs have been generalizations.

Language

NLP suggests these three gatekeepers transform sensory experience into internal representations. They also transform our internal representations when we use language. First we delete, distort and generalize our experience. Then our choice of words to describe the experience deletes, distorts and generalizes it all over again. When we speak, the richness of the original experience is compressed into a linear trickle of words and the whole process takes less time than it takes to read this description. Spoken language, then, is a map of a map and two levels away from sensory experience (see Figure 7.1).

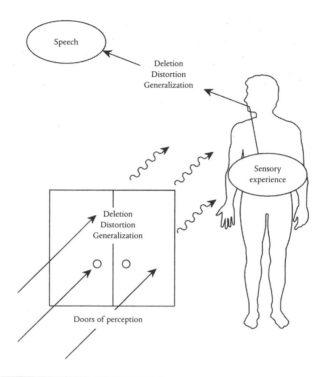

Figure 7.1 Transforming sensory experience to words

The world does not come with labels attached. We attach them and sometimes forget we did so. We can mistake the words we attach to our experience for the experience itself and allow them to direct our actions.

For example, a person decides he does not like 'pop music'. This is a generalization and the words have become a substitute and a barrier to the experience of listening to some types of music. Also we are sometimes fooled by a change of name, thinking that therefore reality has changed. Killing defenceless people is not made any different by calling it 'ethnic cleansing'.

Language does not determine thought, however – it transmits it. Words can be combined in ways that have nothing to do with sensory experience. They free us to express the world of our imagination. This facility is what gives us the freedom to fantasize, to imagine, to discover, to create great works of poetry and literature and move beyond ourselves; to broaden our maps. The danger is in using words to limit and impoverish our maps.

Words do not have a fixed meaning, although we often assume they do. First, very few words have any obvious connection with what they describe. There is nothing 'catlike' about the word 'cat'. Second, words gather meaning from our life experiences. Consequently, the same word can mean different things to different people. Asking a group of people what the word 'love' or 'honour' means will get many different answers. By looking at the words we speak, we can gain some insight into how we delete, distort and generalize experience. Then we can use words to produce a model of the world that is freer, richer and more satisfying. We can 'reverse engineer' the language to get back to the experience.

We can use language in three ways to find out about and influence experience (see Figure 7.2).

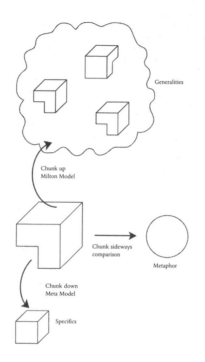

Figure 7.2 Chunking up; chunking down;
chunking sideways

First we can ask questions that connect language with thought and back to sensory experience. This avoids the trap of thinking the word is the experience. For example, someone says to you, 'The people here are unfriendly.' This is a generalization, and we can ask a specific question like, 'Do you mean everybody? Is there no one at all here who is friendly?' This will make the person look at their generalization and see what basis it has in their experience. They will have to look at specific instances. This is called *chunking down* in NLP, going from a general case to more specific ones.

The second way we can use language is to go from specific instances to more general ones. We can use very permissive and vague language that allows the other person to find just that particular meaning that is right for them. (The last sentence was an example of that type of language.) This is called *chunking up*, going from a particular case to a general one.

Finally we can use language to *chunk sideways*: to compare one experience with another. This is the realm of metaphor, simile and story-telling, where you explain, allude or illuminate by comparison. This chapter heading is an example.

Chunking down: language to experience

THE META MODEL

When we use language to chunk down, we are going from the words to the specific experiences that underlie them. We are also discovering how we distort, delete and generalize our experience. To do this, we ask some key questions that follow the thread back through the labyrinth, from the spoken word, past the grammatical structure underlying it to the representational systems and, finally, to sensory experience. The set of questions to accomplish this was the first model developed in NLP by Richard Bandler and John Grinder in 1975 and is called the *Meta Model* (see Bibliography).

To review the Meta Model we will look briefly at the various ways deletion, distortion and generalization translate experience into language, and then at the specific questions we need to ask to reconnect them.

The Meta Model is a series of questions. Some are obvious and we use them without thinking. Others are more subtle. They seek to unravel some of the inevitable selections and distortions in language to clarify communication for both speaker and listener. One way to use the Meta Model is to listen to spoken words and discover what has been left out that would have to be in for the sentence to make sense. What does the listener have to add intuitively? (And maybe guess wrongly?)

DELETIONS

In *Silver Blaze*, one of the cases of Sherlock Holmes, Watson asks: 'Is there any other point to which you wish to draw my attention?'

'To the curious incident of the dog in the night-time,' replies Holmes.

'The dog did nothing in the night-time!'

'That was the curious incident,' remarks Sherlock Holmes.

Like the case of the dog in the night-time, deletions are conspicuous by their absence.

An example:

'People know enough about it.'

What does that sentence mean? It is too vague. We do not know who the people are and it may be important to know exactly who they are. To make sense of it, you would ask, 'What people exactly?'

Sometimes the people are missing completely from a statement – for example, 'Not enough is known about it.' This is called the 'passive voice'. It is a good way of avoiding responsibility, as in the famous government statement, 'Mistakes were made.'

To go back to the original sentence, what does 'it' stand for? Unless that is clear from the previous conversation, you would have to ask, 'What exactly don't they know enough about?' (Even if it seems clear, it is worth asking anyway.)

Finally, the verb 'know' is not very exact. You would have to ask, 'How exactly do they know?'

Conversation would be tedious if we spelled out everything in detail, and every statement has some deletions. However, details can be important. When we don't get them we assume them, often wrongly. *We fill in the missing bits from our maps rather than the speaker's.* Also the speakers themselves may not be clear about what lies behind their statement. Your questions will force them to think back to their actual experience and be more clear about what they mean.

COMPARISONS

The last sentence contained a comparison – 'more'. We use many comparisons: 'better', 'best', 'worse', 'worst', 'more', 'less'. A comparison must involve at least two items.

It may be important to know the basis of the comparison. So you need to ask, 'Compared with what?'

For example, someone says, 'I performed badly.'

Badly compared with what? Your ideal performance? Your performance yesterday? How an expert performs? Unrealistic comparisons guarantee maximum dissatisfaction. One effective way to become depressed and frustrated is to compare yourself with an imaginary and unattainable ideal, feel bad about how far short you are and then delete the standard of comparison you are using. You are then left with a bad feeling and no way to relieve it.

To motivate yourself, compare where you are with an inspiring future, not with other people.

To judge your progress, compare where you are with where you started.

GENERALIZATIONS

The obvious examples here are words like 'all', 'never', 'always' and 'every'. These types of words are called *universals* – they admit no exception. They are limiting, simplifying our view of the world, not the world itself. For example:

'I will never be able to do it.'

'No one cares.'

'You are always out when I need you.'

Sometimes the universals are less obvious. For example:

'People are unkind.'

'French food is expensive.'

'Exceptions prove the rule.'

The way to question these generalizations is to ask for the counter example: 'Are *all* people unkind?' 'Have you never known anyone who was kind?'

Sometimes, if you have good rapport, simply profess incredulity at the statement. '*Never?!*' The speaker then hunts through their experience for exceptions.

Generalizations are also judgements which you may want to question by asking, 'Who says?' or 'What evidence do you have for that statement?' Often we express opinions we no longer really hold. They are left-overs from parental opinions in our early years and need to be dusted off and re-examined.

Another example of generalization is how we set rules for ourselves and others with words like 'ought', 'must', 'should' and 'got to'. These may or may not have good reasons behind them. The way to find out is to ask, 'What would happen if I did not do those things?'

For example, 'You should get another job.'

'What would happen if I didn't?'

Explore the consequences – they may be real and unpleasant or they may be largely imaginary. We are sometimes so mesmerized by these 'ruling' words that we never stop to think but just blindly obey.

There are also the negative rules: 'shouldn't', 'mustn't', 'oughtn't'. To find out the consequences here, ask, 'What would happen if you did?'

For example, 'You mustn't talk to those people.'

'What would happen if I did talk to them?'

Stronger rules are expressed by 'cannot'. Some are clearly physical restraints: 'I can't jump 20 feet.' Others may be beliefs that we have never tested. For example, 'I can't change' or 'I can't find it.' The way round this block is to ask, 'What prevents you?' This changes the focus from being stuck to working towards a goal and eliminating what might stand in your way.

'I can' and 'you can' are empowering phrases (unless they are totally unrealistic). It is a good move to change the 'oughts' and the 'shoulds' to 'cans'.

So, 'I must do well' becomes 'I can do well.' (I probably want to as well and what are the consequences if I do not?)

This replacement is one of the most empowering changes you can make for yourself and others – a simple one-word change.

DISTORTIONS

We distort by taking processes and making them into things. A noun so constructed is called a *nominalization.* Many of our most important concepts are nominalizations: 'love', 'justice', 'education', 'belief', 'choice', 'co-operation', 'fear' and 'memory'. The distortion is that these nouns are really verbs in disguise. A process has become frozen in mid-stride.

The trouble with nominalizations is that they are static and unchangeable. For example, someone says, 'This relationship isn't working.' Find out more about what the speaker means by turning this 'thing' – this relationship – back into a process by asking, 'How exactly are we not *relating*?'

We have already explored statements with parts left out; now here are some distortions that have hidden extras. What is particularly interesting are the assumptions behind what people say. These bring us close to their model of the world. Listen for these assumptions. The way to find them is to ask yourself what else would have to be true for the sentence to make sense.

For example, 'He is as insensitive as your other friends.' This assumes all the other friends are insensitive as well.

'Please do not be as unreasonable as you were last time we discussed this' assumes you were unreasonable and we have discussed the subject before.

'Would you rather pay me now or later?' assumes, of course, that you are going to pay me.

A question beginning with 'why' nearly always hides an assumption by diverting your attention from the assumption to the reason for it.

'Why is this so difficult?' assumes it is difficult in the first place. You actually reinforce the assumption if you answer the 'why' question.

When you seem to be caught in a 'damned if you do and damned if you don't' situation, often called a double bind, rather than thinking you must choose one path or the other, question the assumptions behind the statement. (You might start with the assumption that you *must* choose one or the other.)

Mind-reading is another example of distortion. We may know *how* a person is thinking by watching their eye movements, but we cannot really know *what* they are thinking.

Mind-reading may be a lucky guess or good intuition based on knowing a person well, but it is risky. Why mind-read when you can ask? If someone mind-reads you, ask them exactly how they know what you are thinking.

Adults often profess to mind-read children and tell them what they are or are not feeling. 'Now then, you are not really upset, it's only a game.' It may be only a game, but in the child's world, it is important and they *are* upset. (Adults get upset about games too.)

Some people do 'reverse mind-reading', that is, they assume you can read their mind and therefore should know what they want without being told. This is a confusing pattern if you are on the receiving end.

For example, 'You should know I wanted a holiday.'

How?

Or, even worse, 'If you loved me, you would know I wanted a holiday.'

Now mind-reading is taken as evidence for love!

CAUSE AND EFFECT

Another example of distortion is linking cause and effect in a simplistic way.

Pushing a light switch, for example, 'causes' the light to go on, but obviously this is not the whole story. What we see as cause and effect are merely connections in the material world that we are aware of.

People have choice, unlike inanimate objects, and can react in ways that do not follow the laws of physics. When we make our model of the world we are responsible for the cause–effect links we build in. This is scary and liberating. On the one hand we can no longer blame others for our predicaments. Any problem is at the very least a joint effort between circumstances, other people and self. The liberating part is that if you make your world, you can make it better.

If others are responsible, however, then you are powerless. The English language encourages this way of thinking. 'You bore me' is a way of saying 'You make me feel bored.' Giving other people control over our emotional states is so easy to do with language that we may come to believe it and act as if it were true.

Furthermore, if you act as if you had no choice about your emotional state then the converse also applies: you must be responsible for the emotional states of others. This makes you the victim or the nursemaid of others and can lead to unfounded guilty feelings. (Of course there are always those especially creative individuals who manage to have it both ways: they hold other people responsible for their emotions and expect others to take responsibility for their own emotions.)

There are two ways to question cause and effect.

When you hear 'You make me angry', you can ask, 'How exactly do I make you feel angry?' This asks the speaker to look at their experience. However, they may still just blame you. It is ironic that by doing so, they are putting themselves in the victim role and giving you power over them.

The deeper question is, 'How do you make yourself feel angry in response to what I am doing?' This is a challenging question and disputes the assumption that we are not responsible for our feelings. It advances the idea that we create them in response to other people. Be careful how you use this question.

The Meta Model in practice
The Meta Model has three main uses:

1. It gathers information, by questioning the deletions.

2. It clarifies meaning by asking, 'What do you mean by that?'

3. It identifies limitations, particularly in questioning rules expressed by 'ought' or 'can't', and so opens more choices.

The Meta Model questions also link with the neurological levels mentioned in Chapter 1.

For example, think about the sentence: 'I can't do that here.'

There are a number of ways you might question this statement. What do you choose? That depends on your outcome. Listen to the way the speaker *marks out* what is important with a particular voice tone or gesture, like we *emphasize* words in print.

'I can't do that *here!*' marks out the *environment* level.
You could reply, 'Where could you do it?'

'I can't do *that* here!' marks out the *behaviour* level.
The question to ask now would be, 'What exactly can't you do?' This will question the deletion.

'I can't *do* that here!' marks out the *capability* level.
You could ask, 'What prevents you?' or 'What do you need in order to be able to?'

'I *can't* do that here!' marks out the *belief* level.
You could ask, 'What would happen if you did?' or even 'Why not?'

Finally, '*I* can't do that here!' marks out the *identity* level. The person is saying that they do not feel that they are the sort of person that could do that anywhere. You might ask, 'Who could?'

Use the Meta Model questions when you have rapport, as they can be very challenging. Listen to the other person. What they say reveals their world. Tread lightly into it if you are invited. Repeated questions can seem like a legal cross-examination and some people use these types of specific question only when they are angry. Beware of becoming a Metamonster asking Meta Model questions. Soften the questions by using your voice tone or by asking them in the form of 'I wonder if you would tell me...?' or 'That's interesting, I am not clear about...?'

Applying the Meta Model to yourself: internal dialogue

The best place to apply the Meta Model is to your own internal dialogue.

First you have to listen to it. What exactly are you saying to yourself? For many people, internal dialogue is constant background noise – they do not really listen to it. Listening to the activity of our mind, as a prelude to calming it, can be the basis of meditation. It cleans the doors of perception and starts to chip away at any self-inflicted barriers.

Use the Meta Model questions to find out your own favourite deletions, distortions and generalizations. Discover whether you have any demotivating, unrealistic comparisons in your mind. Listen for outdated judgements – other people's opinions that still echo and emerge instead of a considered answer. Sometimes they come complete with the voice tone of the person they originally belonged to. You may find many 'oughts' and 'can'ts' that unnecessarily limit your freedom of action. And you may catch some of your own beliefs and assumptions and hold them up for a closer look.

Here are some examples:

'I should do this.'
What would happen if you did not?

'I can't do this.'
What stops me?

'He doesn't like me.'
How do I know exactly?

'I'm bored.'
How exactly am I boring myself?

'Change is hard.'
How is changing hard? From what and into what am I changing?

'This decision presents a lot of difficulty.'
How am I finding it difficult deciding?

'No one will help me.'
No one? No one at all?

How and when you apply the Meta Model will depend on your outcome. There will be situations when you are talking to several people at once and you need to speak in a general way so that each individual can make their own meaning of what you say. The next chapter looks at the mirror image of the Meta Model: vague language and what it does.

8

Language, Trance and Stories

We can use language in the opposite way to the Meta Model by chunking up, constructing sentences that offer wide choices of interpretation.

As we have seen, language is very powerful – you cannot not respond to it. When we hear something we have to make some meaning out of it, so we search unconsciously for the way it could be relevant to us. The vaguer it is, the more possible meanings it has.

This is the language of politics. Politics is the art of trying to please everyone all of the time, so typically political announcements are deliberately vague. For example, 'The financial position is greatly improved, unemployment is down and we look forward to being able to consider a modest decrease in taxation.' This does not tell you the financial position at the moment or how it is measured. Unemployment may be slightly down from a very high level or the rules about how it is measured may have changed. The sort of taxation or what decrease, if any, is not specified. If disappointment requires enhanced expectation, then politicians should not be surprised at the disappointment they generate.

The other place we find this vague language is paradoxically in popular songs. Most pop songs are about love and relationships and they must have universal appeal.

Most do not give any time or place for action and they could equally be sung by either sex and still make sense.

The Milton Model

NLP has studied this type of language, calling it the *Milton Model*. The Milton Model is the mirror image of the Meta Model; it is a way of constructing sentences that are rife with deletions, distortions and generalizations. It originated from the modelling work done by Richard Bandler and John Grinder on Milton Erickson's artfully vague use of language (see Bibliography).

Milton Erickson was one of the foremost hypnotherapists of the twentieth century. A client goes to a therapist because they cannot solve their problem consciously on their own. The resources they need are unconscious. Erickson used language firstly to pace and lead the person's reality. He described their ongoing sensory experience in very general terms and then led them deeper into their own internal reality. He used complex language to distract their conscious mind and allow access to the unconscious resources. When the client was in a trance, Erickson enabled them to search for the resources they needed from their unconscious with vague, open, permissive language and metaphors.

To get a sense of this general language, relax for a moment as you continue reading this paragraph, and begin to think of all the possibilities of this type of language, of the times when it is right to use it, and the times it is right to use specific language, and begin to consider that perhaps you have always known this and used it without giving it any thought, so you can easily let your unconscious mind continue to think exactly how and when you could use these language patterns in your life, so you can pleasantly surprise yourself with the realization that you have more skill than you were consciously aware of.

Trance

So the Milton Model originated in hypnotherapy and was used to induce trance. Trance is not a special state evoked only by skilled hypnotists after much concentration. It is a naturally occurring state that we slip in and out of all the time, and is essential for mental health. Our attention is always somewhere between being focused completely outwards on the outside world with minimal awareness of ourselves or being focused on our internal world. Trance is a state where our attention is tightly focused on our internal world, and any language pattern that increases our involvement with our own internal reality will deepen the trance.

Trance affects groups of people. Audiences at a concert, rock or classical, are in a shared trance, so are crowds at a football match. Groups of people at rallies or listening to inspirational speakers or at religious ceremonies go into a trance. People who have been in a disaster such as a fire or earthquake or who have been attacked are 'numb' or 'shell-shocked'. This is a kind of trance state. It is important for authorities who deal with these disasters to realize this and restore the people to a resourceful state as quickly as possible.

What part does trance play in everyday life? More than you might expect. Have you ever been in a meeting where you were sort of listening to the speaker, but you 'spaced out' for a moment? When you are watching television you are in a sort of trance – your attention is fixed on one point and you are 'gone' from the rest of the world. People may call your name and get no response, even though your ears are working normally. On other occasions there is some external distraction and you 'snap out' of your reverie. Next time you are in a lift or in a railway carriage, notice the glassy-eyed expressions on the faces of your fellow travellers. They have retreated into their internal world and are in a light trance. Notice how they 'wake up' at their station.

The traditional signs of trance to look for are: body immobility, relaxed face, slowing reflexes, time distortion, feeling distanced or dissociated. However, it need not be exactly so; for example, a computer game is a very effective trance inducer.

Day-dreaming is a form of trance, usually a very creative one. When you day-dream, you are open to ideas from your unconscious. Many scientific breakthroughs happen this way – inventors report the solution came to them in a flash as they were deeply immersed in the problem. One of the great discoveries in physics – the general theory of relativity – was made by a young scientist called Albert Einstein imagining what it would be like to ride on the end of a light beam.

Everyday trances

Rather than give a more detailed description of the Milton Model, we would like to look at trance in everyday life and the practical applications that follow. Suppose life were a series of trances, some deep, some shallow, some short, others long lasting. Some of these everyday trances we have control over – we can 'snap out' of them. Others catch and hold us. Some are productive and creative. You can see children going into a trance as you describe Christmas and tell them of the parties and presents. They are imagining what it will be like. They have gone into the future, creating, anticipating and drawing on memories of the past. They are wide-eyed, enjoying a pleasant and positive trance. A historical romance, science fiction or horror story, if it is well written, will transport us to an imaginary world. Most of us have gone to bed after reading a horror story or seeing a frightening film and pulled the covers over our head to keep out the monsters. The imaginary world can invade the real one.

Here is an example of a negative trance. Joseph was doing some consulting work for a company. His contact at the company called him and questioned the results, expressed dissatisfaction and suggested that perhaps the fee was too high. He came off the telephone and started to think about all the times when he was at school and people had questioned his work unfairly. He thought about what he had done for that company. He was sure it was good work and had dealt with the important issues. Perhaps they would not pay him! He became indignant. How dare they! It was really unfair! They had no right. He nearly marched into the next meeting ready to tell them they could keep their wretched money and he didn't want to work with the company any more, thank you very much. This was his trance. In fact his contact had reviewed the situation and was satisfied. The cheque was in the post that day.

What are your everyday trances? Are there any unresourceful trances you repeatedly find yourself in? Find out what triggers them. It could be external, for example a particular critical tone of voice. It could be internal, a particular thought or memory. Trance triggers are like trapdoors – once you have fallen through, it is very difficult to get back. Catch the trance before it develops and do not associate into it. If you find you are in it, then acknowledge that and come out by focusing on the external world. When you are in the present moment, you are not in a trance. Remember the trance is not you. It is something you go into and so it is something you can come out of.

All our trances have some purpose – they are attempts to solve problems. Think about what the trance does for you. Respect the intention and change the behaviour.

Metaphor

Metaphor is halfway between the unintelligible and the commonplace.

(Aristotle)

Metaphor is used in NLP to cover figures of speech, stories, comparisons, similes and parables. Metaphors chunk sideways from one thing to another, making comparisons and connections that may be subtle or obvious. To make sense of our experience we need to make comparisons. Put the tips of your fingers on the surface nearest you and notice the information you get about it through your sense of touch. Now run your fingers slowly along it. Now you are getting many different touches and by comparing them you know much more of the character of the surface, its texture and temperature.

Stories are our birthright and metaphors pervade our thinking. They are woven into our lives at every level, from the bedtime stories we listened to as children to the ways we think about work, life, relationships and health. They build creative connections between two events or experiences, giving another, different, hopefully illuminating example. Religious teachers speak in metaphors and parables, paradoxically to make their ideas clearer.

Take an example:

Life is like...

How would you complete this and what would that mean?

Is life a bowl of cherries? A struggle? An adventure? A school? A test? A vale of tears? A wheel? A jungle?

The metaphors a person uses give the key to their life and the way they think. A person to whom life is an adventure is going to approach events quite differently from a person for whom life is a struggle.

Organizations use metaphors. An organization that prides itself on its team players is going to react differently from one that sees itself as a fighting force. One current metaphor for business is 'a learning organization', which conjures up a rather different picture. Some organizations still call themselves 'family businesses', a powerful metaphor of what they stand for and the way they treat their employees.

Strangely, the financial world is sprinkled with liquid metaphors. They talk of cash flow, flooding the market, liquid and frozen assets, floating a company. Money is like water, perhaps?

The world of selling is *armed* with metaphors. Many sales books and trainings describe selling as a battle – the customer is the enemy and objections must be attacked. Such courses are like military academies. Sometimes sales books talk of wooing the customer or seducing them, others of chipping away at objections like a sculptor with a chisel. The metaphor the salesperson carries is going to affect how they approach and deal with the customer.

Health and medicine, too, are full of metaphors, not all of them healthy. We talk of the 'war against cancer', 'fighting illness' and 'eradicating germs'. Our immune system, our identity on the physiological level, is likened to a killing machine. If it is efficient, then we are healthy. If it 'breaks down', then we will fall ill. Other, perhaps more helpful metaphors of health are to do with balance, working with the body and co-existence.

Metaphors are not right or wrong, but they have consequences for how people think and act – consequences which are implicit in the metaphor.

Problem-solving

In metaphors, people and experiences do not have to be one thing or the other: they can be both or neither. One and one does not always equal two. One and one can equal one if they are raindrops. One and one equals nil if they are black holes, and one plus one can equal three when two people are in love.

Think of a current difficult situation in your life. Think of your problem as a short metaphor. Quickly. Your problem is like…

A jam doughnut? A ringing telephone? A poker game? A fight with a dragon?

This is your present state.

Now look at your metaphor. What are the assumptions inherent in that metaphor? What else would have to be true for that metaphor to be accurate?

Now think of what you would prefer the problem to be like. Quickly make another metaphor. You would prefer…

Now think how the problem is like that.

What are the differences between the first metaphor and the second metaphor? How could you get from one to the other? How are they similar? The connection could be the resource that helps you from one to the other.

Milton Erickson used to tell stories to his clients. The starting-point would be in some way similar to the client's problem. The end would be in some way a resolution. The connection between the two would be the resource needed to solve the problem.

Giving people instructions about what they 'should' do does not work. They know already, but it is just conscious mind information. A metaphor goes beyond conscious understanding.

For example, Ian was working with a married couple who were experiencing some difficulties in their relationship. Although basically they wanted to stay together, they found it difficult to co-operate. Ian tasked them to take dancing lessons together. Both had learned to dance a little in the past, but not with each other. Dancing was a metaphor for their relationship. As they learned to dance together, they physically learned the give and take, ebb and flow, lead and follow that they had lacked in their relationship. Metaphors are very powerful in relationships; the ones we have influence how we treat our partners. For example, marriage could be a battle of the sexes, a joining, a sacred vow or a peaceful co-existence.

Systems of psychology use metaphors that are very revealing. The 'subconscious' of psychoanalysis, for example, sounds murkier than the unconscious, because the prefix 'sub' means underneath, as in subterranean and subhuman. Underneath is a metaphor for inferior or bad – the heavens are above and hell beneath. Gestalt has a 'top dog' and an 'underdog'. Transactional Analysis is full of metaphor. People have parts – the adult, the inner child, the little professor – and there is the idea of a 'life script'.

What metaphor are you living? A tale of self-sacrifice? An heroic quest? What sort of film would it make? A comedy or a tragedy?

Once upon a time...

We need stories. They are so important that we tell ourselves half a dozen in our sleep every night, although we do not always remember them. These dreams often seem strange to our conscious mind, yet they are often very creative. Stories are so much part of our everyday life, we sometimes forget their power.

We come home from work or school and turn on the television to be confronted by – stories. Journalists know that even the news is a story. Have you heard them say, 'And the top news story today is...'?

All our technology still delivers us stories. William Gibson, the science fiction writer who coined the word 'cyberspace' in his novel *Neuromancer*, wrote a book some years ago that you could access online. As you read it on the screen it self-destructed – a metaphor perhaps for the ephemeral nature of digital information. The computer itself is often taken as a metaphor for the brain. If the brain *is* like a computer, then who has programmed it?

Gregory Bateson, the British writer who influenced NLP at its inception, tells a story in his book *Steps to an Ecology of Mind*. It concerns a man who wanted to know the real nature of the mind, how far a computer was a good model for a brain and whether, as the power of computers increased, they would ever be as intelligent as humans. He typed a question into the most powerful contemporary computer: 'Do you compute that you will ever think like a human being?'

The machine whirred and stuttered as it put the question through its circuits, trying to analyse its own method of analysing. Eventually, it printed its reply.

The man bounded over to see what the computer had typed. He read, 'That reminds me of a story...'

9

Beliefs and Beyond

Beliefs

Beliefs have us. They drive our behaviour. They are intangible and frequently unconscious. They are often confused with facts. But while a fact is what happened, a belief is a generalization about what will happen. It is a guiding principle.

We share certain beliefs about the physical world based on facts. For example, fire burns and we are subject to the laws of gravity, so we do not tempt fate by walking off cliffs or by holding live electric cables. However, we have many beliefs about ourselves and other people that control our behaviour just as effectively as the belief that fire burns, and these may or may not be true. It is these beliefs that NLP is interested in.

When people tell you they believe something, they are either telling you of a value they hold dear or their best guess in the absence of knowledge. Beliefs answer the question 'Why?'

The generalizations which form beliefs are justified in one of two ways. The first is by linking cause and effect, the second comes from making meaning.

Cause and effect

'I don't understand computers because I have never been taught.'

'I am insecure because my family moved around a lot when I was young.'

'I am creative because I am a Leo.'

These examples link an experience in the present with a presumed cause in the past. However, causal connections are tricky when you are dealing with complex events, as we have to take so much for granted, and fallacies abound. A connection is not a cause. For example, statistics show video rentals have increased in line with the population increase, but they are somehow unlikely to have caused it.

Such cause–effect links cannot be proven, but they give a reason, and it is important for us to have reasons to make sense of our experience. Some belief is better than no belief and this is why people can take grim satisfaction out of calamity, provided they had predicted it. Beliefs make sense of the world, they give coherence to our experience. This is so whether the belief is supportive or undermining. Beliefs help us navigate the future and protect the present.

Meaning

Second, beliefs give meaning to experiences by connecting them.

For example:

'If you are ill it *means* you have not taken care of yourself.'

'If you cannot give up smoking it *means* you have no will-power.'

'If someone loves me this *means* I am a lovable person.'

Again these connections can be argued but not proven. They came from the speaker's map of the world.

What we believe about others determines how we treat them and so, in turn, their response to us. For example, a person who believes other people are basically untrustworthy will be suspicious of others and their motives. This will make others wary of them, which will reinforce their original belief. Beliefs act as self-fulfilling prophecies. When we treat someone as if they are capable and intelligent, they are likely to become so. What we believe filters our experience. We take notice of instances that confirm our beliefs and delete counter-examples, unless they are particularly striking. Reason does not form our beliefs, so you cannot argue a person out of them with conventional logic.

Submodalities and beliefs

Beliefs have a submodality structure. A belief is coded with one set of submodalities, doubt with another.

Think of something you believe implicitly. For example, the sun will rise tomorrow. Make a picture that expresses that belief and include sounds and feelings. Do not confuse the feeling *about* the picture (that it is convincing and you believe it) with any feelings that are *part of* the picture. The convincing feeling is your response to the visual and auditory submodalities.

Now think of something you doubt. Make a picture to express that doubt.

Look at your two pictures – one of belief, one of doubt. The content of the pictures will be different, of course, and the submodalities of the two pictures will be different too. We each have a personal submodality structure of what we believe.

Belief formation

Beliefs are formed haphazardly throughout life from the meaning we give to our experience. They are formed during our upbringing from modelling significant others, especially our parents. They can be formed from a sudden unexpected conflict, trauma or confusion, and the younger we are, the more likely this is to happen. Sometimes beliefs are formed by repetition – the experience has no emotional intensity, but it just keeps happening, like water dripping on a stone.

Because children do not have the experience and knowledge that come from living, they can make some unexpected connections. Joseph's five-year-old daughter once asked him if she had to break an arm or leg to become an adult. This seemed a strange question until he realized that she actually knew a number of people who had broken a bone in their teens. A friend had broken a leg in a car accident that week and the preceding day Joseph had told her how he had broken his arm when he was 14.

Empowering and limiting beliefs

Some of our beliefs give us freedom, choice and open possibilities. Others may be disempowering, closing down choice. Acting as if they were true makes you and others miserable.

Beliefs are often expressed in the form:

'I can...'

'I can't...'

'I shouldn't...'

'I must...'

Take a moment to write down some examples you have of each of those four.

Do you get the sense that those that start 'I can't...' and 'I shouldn't...' limit your choices? Examine them using the Meta Model. Ask yourself, 'What prevents me?' and 'What would happen if I did?' Even beliefs that begin 'I must...' may be problematic if you feel that this is so under *all* circumstances.

Belief change

Do you believe that it is possible to change your beliefs? Would you like to change some? After all, it makes sense to have some empowering ones that make life a pleasure.

You have already changed beliefs in the past. You do not believe now what you did when you were five years old. As we grow and gain experience, our beliefs change, although we do not always notice. Sometimes a belief can be destroyed by one powerful exception. This leaves a vacuum into which any belief may fall, however strange, and this can be the basis of dramatic conversions.

When you change a belief we suggest you replace it with another belief that keeps the positive intention of the old one. The new one must also be congruent with your sense of self.

To change a negative belief you need to ask yourself, 'What is this belief doing for me?' and 'What belief would I rather have?'

There are some good questions you can ask yourself before you consider changing any belief you have:

'How will my life be better with the new belief?'

'How might my life be worse with the new belief?'

'What is the best thing that could happen if I kept the old belief?'

'What is the best thing that could happen with the new belief?'

Belief changes may not last if you give up too soon. For example, someone wants to play a better game of tennis. They find a good coach and start to believe they will improve with a new technique. They stop using their old technique and begin to learn a new way, but because it is unfamiliar, paradoxically their results are worse. With a better technique, they will improve in time, but they may become discouraged too soon, revert to the old method and then believe that they cannot improve.

NLP has a number of techniques for changing limiting beliefs. Some work by changing the submodality structures of the old and new beliefs. Another involves going back to the imprint experience that generated the belief and re-evaluating it from a resourceful position. Whatever the technique, it is important that the new belief fits with the person's values and sense of self.

Beliefs and health

The influence of our beliefs on our health is one of the clearest examples of the mind and body being one system. The medical profession has tremendous credibility. We believe what doctors tell us. A drastic one-sentence belief change would be a doctor's diagnosis of cancer. Such a sentence (in both senses of the word) is an example of the power of belief and some people will literally die of the diagnosis. Deepak Chopra, in his book *Quantum Healing* (Bantam 1989), gives many examples of the effect of both life-enhancing and life-denying beliefs and their effects on health. Beliefs and health is a really important and fascinating area where there is tremendous scope for useful practical applications.

Another example of belief and health is the 'placebo effect' – a significant minority of patients cure themselves if they believe they are being given an effective drug, even when they are being given an inert substance with no curative effect. Drugs will not always work, while belief in recovery is always useful and sometimes essential.

Belief and action

As already mentioned, beliefs drive behaviour. Sometimes we hold conflicting beliefs and then we will be incongruent. Sometimes people profess to believe in a particular value, but their behaviour contradicts it. Behaviour is belief in action, whatever we may consciously say we believe.

We generalize most of our beliefs, making them true or false in all contexts. Need this be so? As we have already seen, in NLP you can choose your beliefs. They are maps of reality. When we believe something we act as if it were true, but that does not make it true. Nor does it make it false. It will be true for you in that moment.

To understand the effect of beliefs, choose the ones you want carefully. Choose those that give you the life you wish for.

The final principle of NLP we want to address is one that makes all the others real:

If you want to understand – act.

Because the learning is in the doing. Principles make a difference in action.

For example, we hold core beliefs about our identity that have profound effects. 'I am basically a good person who makes mistakes sometimes' and 'I am a stupid person who sometimes gets it right by luck' will give very different experiences.

We also have beliefs about what lies beyond our identity. When Albert Einstein was asked what was the most important question for mankind to ask, he replied, 'The most important question facing humanity is: Is the Universe a friendly place?'

How we answer that question brings us to what it means to be a person and that takes us into the spiritual realm.

NLP and spirituality

What a piece of work is a man! How noble in reason! How infinite in faculty! In form and moving, how express and admirable! In action, how like an angel! In apprehension, how like a god! The beauty of the world! The paragon of animals!

(William Shakespeare,
Hamlet, Act III, v. 316)

Throughout history people have searched, driven by the feeling that 'we see through a glass darkly', and that there is more to life than body and mind. We are constantly reaching out beyond ourselves to know by experience our connection and unity with that which is more than ourselves. What can NLP contribute?

NLP deals with the structure of human experience and so these major issues are very much in its province. We are also personally drawn to exploring them with NLP. Were NLP to be silent about spiritual experience, then it could give the message that spiritual experience is somehow different and removed from life. This is not so.

NLP itself makes no claim on reality, truth, morality or ethics. It treats these as subjective experiences. It does not acknowledge or deny an external reality, but simply suggests you act as if the presuppositions are true and notice the results you get. NLP asks not 'Is it true?' but 'Is it useful?'

How you decide what you want and how you will achieve it are ethical and moral questions. How can we use the utility of NLP in the service of ethics and aesthetics? These are necessarily the responsibility of the NLP practitioner: we each apply our own morality and ethics to both our outcomes and the means we choose to achieve them. The basis for the ethics is our common humanity and our deepest essence as human beings.

Spirituality could be said to be about finding our basic humanity – the same essence we share with every person. And in discovering that, we are finding still more. Words fall short of spiritual experience like stones thrown at the stars. One way of thinking of it is as a feeling of being most truly ourselves and in the process discovering and becoming most deeply connected with others in their full magnificence. There are moments like this in most people's lives. You do not have to spend a lifetime of prayer, mortification and self-denial to have them. Some religious traditions hold that spiritual experiences are hard to come by, but they are all around – those splashes of joy and insight that can happen at any time, those peak experiences when you feel most fully alive. Giving birth and becoming a parent, feeling your connection with life, looking into the eyes of a newborn child, these can all be spiritual experiences.

What has been your spiritual experience? Take a moment to remember those times in your life when you felt most fully yourself and most fully connected with others. Keep those experiences in mind as you read on.

A universal metaphor for spiritual experience is a search, quest or journey, and the end of our search, in the words of T. S. Eliot in 'The Four Quartets', will be to 'arrive where we started and know the place for the first time'. The answers on the outside are mirrored within us. Or, as Gertrude Stein put it, "There never has been an answer, there never will be an answer – that's the answer.'

Modelling spiritual experience

NLP can be used to model spiritual experience both in self and others. We have models, we have writings and we have experience. NLP approaches spirituality through individual experience, not organized religion. It looks for a similar structure to spiritual experiences, regardless of whether they are Christian, Jewish, Taoist, Buddhist or any other.

How can we start to look at spiritual experience, how can we model it? Human life is a series of separations followed by integration – we are continually knowing ourselves more fully by knowing what we are *not*... A child is born and separates from the mother, and with growing self-awareness begins to separate their identity from the world and other people. There is a growing realization of individuality. The child establishes a first position: 'I am me. You are you. We are not the same.'

The adolescent has a further task: to separate from the confines of the family and participate in the wider world. Then as adults we need to develop a strong sense of self, to know and value ourselves as unique individuals, for without this step we cannot continue the spiritual journey.

Having achieved independence, we are ready to explore interdependence. You cannot go beyond the ego unless you have developed one in the first place. A spiritual journey is paradoxical in the sense you are continually developing aspects of yourself in order to go beyond them. Unless you develop them, you cannot transcend them. We come to know ourselves by constantly finding out what we are not.

We are not our behaviour, we are not our capabilities, we are not our beliefs. We are not even our identity. What are we?

What practical help is NLP in this quest?

Acting on the principles of NLP builds a strong sense of self. You become more self-aware by paying attention and becoming curious about your own experience in a non-judgemental way. Personal change and development become a natural process rather than a hard struggle, something you only do at special times and places. Where you are right now is exactly the right place, and what you have are exactly the right resources to move on. What you do at any one time may not seem important, but it is very important that you do it.

Setting outcomes gives congruence and clarity about what you want. As you begin to pace yourself, you become less divided, more relaxed and intuitive, more congruent and in harmony. Many spiritual writings speak of the world and the self as a process. NLP suggests that 'I' is a nominalization. The ego is not a fixed thing, but a dynamic process, a principle of action. Even the body that seems so permanent is in a state of flux. We are a river, not a statue. The skin renews itself every month. We have a new liver every six weeks, a new skeleton every three months. Ninety eight per cent of the atoms in your body were not there one year ago.

The Meta Model can show the deletions, distortions and generalizations that limit our world. When we use it on our internal dialogue, we can begin to know what sort of inner conversationalist we are. Internal dialogue is one of the principal ways we limit ourselves by continually reinforcing our identification with our behaviour, likes and dislikes, and even with the dialogue itself. The Meta Model, together with choosing our anchors, can begin to break the cause–effect triggers between action and reaction and lead to an experience of real choice about our emotional state. It also clarifies how our language is shaping our experience. How we talk about something does not define it. It is particularly difficult to talk about the spiritual. It has to be through metaphor. Language separates this from that, light from darkness. It deals in opposites. The spiritual is about connection, where it is possible to be both at once, or neither.

NLP alerts us to our presuppositions and beliefs. It helps by bringing us to our senses, by giving the tools and opportunities to come out of any life-debilitating trances we may be caught in. NLP looks both ways: outside to the world of the senses and inside to our subjective experience. It can bring us into the present moment by directing our attention to what we actually see, hear and feel rather than our interpretations.

We do have to engage in the world – spiritual experience is found by engaging fully in life, fully committing, even in the face of adversity and impermanence.

There has also to be a balance between the conscious and unconscious mind. In Western culture, there is a danger of too much reliance on the conscious mind. But we cannot consciously predict what will happen nor control the world. This need not lead to giving up, but to knowing our conscious limits. The only thing to give up is the illusion of control, where the conscious mind takes responsibility and credit for everything that happens. In fact, the conscious mind sets the direction and the unconscious moves. The conscious mind is like the rider who sets the course but should not try to tell the horse exactly where to put its feet. The horse needs guidance. So building rapport, a resourceful relationship, with your unconscious is a profound thing to do. It has great spiritual importance. NLP provides the means for doing this.

The separation of behaviour from intention is another crucial principle. It goes naturally with the realization that we are not our behaviour and enables us to sense our common humanity. This does not excuse nor condone the dreadful actions that humanity is capable of: recognition is not justification.

NLP alerts us to our beliefs and presuppositions. What is our normal state? Is it one of suffering, of trying, of struggle against desire? Is our life metaphor one of struggle? What do we presuppose about human beings? Are they basically flawed and not to be trusted? Are they alright sometimes? Or are they incredible, magnificent and acting with purpose driven by a positive intention, even when behaving destructively, mistakenly and unconsciously?

Positive intention cannot be proved. Neither can the opposite. But we do have a choice about the presuppositions we operate from. Some will make for a fulfilling life.

The last part of the spiritual journey is going beyond oneself to what we really are, in our deepest nature. Whatever reality is, our maps will only give us knowledge *about* it. To know it *directly* we have to experience it. The metaphor of the spiritual quest very often ends with the person finding within what they were looking for outside. They thought they did not have it, but then they realize that they had it all along without knowing. Whatever reality is, it cannot be external or internal, it just is. Both. We must be part of reality. We are so much part of it that we cannot see it; it is like trying to see inside our own eyes. The conscious mind tends to be dualistic – things are either this or that – so it has a hard time grasping this point. The moment it tries to do so, it separates from the experience and there is nothing to grasp. Our conscious mind cannot see the whole picture unless it is engaged with all of us, including that which is other-than-conscious.

Our representational systems and our senses make only maps, and the map is not the territory. However, that does not mean we have to give them up. Our senses connect us with the world outside our skin. What are their equivalents that connect us directly with the world within? One answer could be meditation. Certain kinds of meditation have measurable effects on the nervous system, giving a paradoxical state of restful alertness (see Appendix 3).

By modelling spiritual experience, NLP helps you track its footprints down to the river. Once you are there you can decide whether you want to pause or take the plunge.

A final story from the Chinese master Chuang Tzu. Someone had told him his words were useless.

Chuang Tzu said, 'A man has to understand the useless before you can talk to him about the useful. The earth is certainly vast and broad, though a man uses no more of it than the area he puts his feet on. If, however, you were to dig away all the earth he was not standing on, then would the man still be able to make use of it?'

'No, it would be useless' was the reply.

'It is obvious then', said Chuang Tzu, 'that the useless has its uses.'

Appendix 1

PRESUPPOSITIONS OF NLP

The principles of NLP are called presuppositions because you presuppose them to be true and then act. It is not claimed that they are true or universal. However, in our experience, if you act as if they were true you will find your life and interactions with others become more effective, interesting, satisfying and enriching.

There is no orthodox list of NLP presuppositions. We have selected the ones that are most commonly used and which we think are the most important.

- **People respond to their map of reality and not to reality itself.**

  We operate and communicate from those maps. NLP is the art of changing these maps, not reality.

- **Human behaviour is purposeful.**

  We are not always conscious of what that purpose is.

- **All behaviour has a positive intention.**

  Our behaviour is always trying to achieve something valuable for us. A person is not their behaviour. NLP separates the intention or purpose behind an action from the action itself. What appears as negative behaviour is only so because we do not see the purpose.

- **The unconscious mind is benevolent.**

  The unconscious mind balances the conscious; it is not inherently malevolent.

- **Having choice is better than not having choice.**

  Seek a map for yourself that makes the widest and richest number of choices available. Act always to increase choice. The person with the most number of choices, that is, the greatest flexibility of thought and behaviour, will have the greatest influence in any interaction.

- **People make the best choice they can at the time.**

  No matter how self-defeating, bizarre or evil the behaviour, it is the best choice available to that person at that time, given their map of the world. Give them a better choice in their map of the world and they will take it.

- **People work perfectly.**

  No one is wrong or broken. It is a matter of finding out how they function, so that it can effectively be changed to something more useful and desirable.

- **The meaning of the communication is the response you get.**

  This may be different from the one you intended. There are no failures in communication, only responses and feedback. Every experience can be utilized. If you are not getting the result you want, do something different.

- **We either already have all the resources we need or we can create them.**

  There are no unresourceful people, only unresourceful states.

- **The mind and body are one system.**

  They interact and mutually influence each other. It is not possible to make a change in one without the other being affected.

- **We process all information through our senses.**

  Take away a human being's capacity to sense and you take away their ability to experience the external world.

- **Modelling successful performance leads to excellence. If one person can do something it is possible to model it and teach it to others.**

  Excellence can be duplicated.

- **If you want to understand – act.**

  The learning is in the doing.

Appendix 2

GLOSSARY

accessing cues The ways we tune our bodies by breathing, posture, gesture and eye movements to think in certain ways.

anchor Any stimulus that evokes a response. Anchors can change our *state*.

anchoring The process of associating one thing with another. *Anchors* can occur naturally or be set up intentionally.

associated state Inside an experience, seeing through your own eyes, fully in your senses.

behaviour Any activity that we engage in, including thought processes. One of the *neurological levels*.

beliefs The *generalizations* we make about ourselves, others and the world, and our operating principles in it. One of the *neurological levels*.

body language The way we communicate with our body, without words or sounds. For example, our posture, gestures, facial expressions, appearance and *accessing cues*.

calibration Accurately recognizing another person's *state* by reading non-verbal signals.

capability A successful *strategy* for carrying out a task. A skill. One of the *neurological levels*.

chunking Changing your perception by going up or down a level. The *Meta Model* chunks down from language by asking for specific instances. The *Milton Model* chunks up from language by including a number of possible specific instances in a general phrase structure.

congruence   Alignment of *beliefs*, values, skills and action. Being in *rapport* with oneself.

conscious   Anything in present-moment awareness.

cross-over matching   *Matching* a person's *body language* with a different type of movement, for example tapping your foot in time to their speech rhythm.

deletion   In speech or thought, missing out a portion of an experience.

dissociated state   Being at one remove from an experience, seeing or hearing it from the outside.

distortion   Changing experience, making it different in some way.

environment   The where and the when and the people we are with. One of the *neurological levels*.

eye accessing cues   Movements of the eyes in certain directions which indicate visual, auditory or *kinaesthetic* thinking.

first position   Perceiving the world from your own point of view only. Being in touch with your own inner reality.

generalization   The process by which one specific experience comes to represent a whole class of experiences.

identity   Your self-image or self-concept. Who you take yourself to be. One of the *neurological levels*.

in time   Having a *timeline* where the past is behind you and the future in front, with the 'now' part passing through your body.

incongruence   *State* of being out of *rapport* with oneself, having internal conflict expressed in *behaviour*. It may be sequential – for example, one action followed by another that contradicts it – or simultaneous – for example, agreement in words but with a doubtful voice tone.

kinaesthetic   The feeling sense, tactile sensations and internal feelings such as remembered sensations, emotions and the sense of balance.

lead system   The *representational system* you use to access stored information: for example, for some people a mental picture of a holiday scene will bring back the whole experience.

leading   Changing what you do with enough *rapport* for the other person to follow.

map of reality   Each person's unique representation of the world built from their individual perceptions and experiences.

matching   Adopting parts of another person's *behaviour*, skills, beliefs or values for the purpose of enhancing *rapport*.

Meta Model   A model of language which is based on the use of universal *modelling* principles. A set of language patterns and questions that link language with experience.

metaphor   Indirect communication by a story or figure of speech implying a comparison. In NLP 'metaphor' covers similes, stories, parables and allegories.

Milton Model   The inverse of the *Meta Model*, using artfully vague language patterns to pace another person's experience and access *unconscious resources*.

mismatching   Adopting different patterns of *behaviour* from another person for the purpose of redirecting, interrupting or ending either your interaction with them (as in a meeting or conversation) or their way of relating to themselves.

modelling   The process of discerning the sequence of ideas and *behaviour* that enables someone to accomplish a task. The basis of NLP.

multiple description   The wisdom of having different points of view of the same event. There are three perceptual positions. *First position*: your own reality; *second position*: another person's reality; and *third position*: a detached viewpoint. Having all three is called a multiple description.

neuro-linguistic programming   The study of excellence, a model of how individuals structure their experience and the study of the structure of subjective experience.

neurological levels   Different levels of experience: *environment, behaviour, capability, beliefs, identity* and *spiritual.*

nominalization   Linguistic term for the process of turning a verb into an abstract noun; also the word for the noun so formed. For example, 'relating' becomes 'the relationship': a process has become a thing.

outcome   A specific, sensory-based, desired goal. You know what you will see, hear and feel when you have it.

pacing   Gaining and maintaining *rapport* with another person over a period of time by meeting them in their model of the world.

positive intention   The positive purpose underlying any action or belief.

predicates   Sensory-based words that indicate the use of one *representational system.*

preferred representational system   The *representational system* that an individual typically uses most to think consciously and organize his or her experience.

presuppositions   Ideas or *beliefs* that are presupposed, that is, taken for granted and acted upon.

rapport   A relationship of trust and responsiveness with self or others.

representational system   The different channels whereby we re-present information on the inside, using our senses: visual (sight), auditory (hearing), *kinaesthetic* (body sensation), olfactory (smell) and gustatory (taste).

resources   Anything that can help you achieve an *outcome*, for example physiology, *states*, thoughts, *beliefs*, strategies, experiences, people, events, possessions, places, stories, etc.

second position   Seeing the world from another person's point of view and so understanding their reality to some extent.

self-modelling   *Modelling* your own *states* of excellence as *resources.*

sensory acuity   The process of learning to make finer and more useful distinctions from the sense information we get from the world.

spiritual   That level of experience where you are most yourself and most your Self and you are most connected with others. One of the *neurological levels.*

state   The sum of our thoughts, feelings, emotions and physical and mental energy

strategy   A repeatable sequence of thought and *behaviour* which consistently produces a particular *outcome.*

submodalities   The fine distinctions we make within each *representational system,* the qualities of our internal representations, the smallest building blocks of our thoughts.

third position   Perceiving the world from the viewpoint of a detached observer.

timeline   The line that connects your past with your future. The way we store pictures, sounds and feelings of our past, present and future.

trance   An altered *state* resulting from a temporarily fixed, narrowed and inward focus of attention.

unconscious   Everything that is not in your present-moment awareness.

Appendix 3

MEDITATION

Many kinds of meditation are currently available. We can make a distinction between 'stick' and 'carrot' approaches. The first kind depends on concentration, requiring focused attention to the exclusion of other external stimuli, for example concentration on a candle flame. In our opinion, such approaches are not always effective because they do not utilize the brain's natural way of functioning. (You can spend a lot of time trying not to notice anything other than the candle flame.) We know that when our surroundings are not stimulating, our minds seek out more pleasing experiences and will generate internal experience of their own. We also know that one thought triggers another by association.

The second kind of meditative approach harnesses this tendency of the mind to move to greater satisfaction, stimulation and happiness, and as a result does not require any forced concentration. The great advantage of this approach is that it works in the same way as your mind works and does not require you to strain. Essentially, it charms the mind to experience itself more fully and more profoundly.

BIBLIOGRAPHY

A selection of classic works:

Andreas, Connirae and Andreas, Steve, *Heart of the Mind*, Real People Press, 1989.
A book that gives many strategies based around submodalities.

Bandler, Richard, *Using Your Brain for a Change*, Real People Press, 1985.
A wide-ranging introduction to submodalities in NLP.

Bandler, Richard, and Grinder, John, *Patterns of the Hypnotic Techniques of Milton H. Erickson M.D. Volume 1*, Meta Publications, 1975.
The results of the modelling work by Bandler and Grinder with Milton Erickson. A detailed model of the artfully vague language patterns known as the Milton Model.

Bandler, Richard, and Grinder, John, *The Structure of Magic 1*, Science and Behaviour Books, 1975.
A full description of the Meta Model. The first NLP book published.

Bateson, Gregory, *Steps to an Ecology of Mind*, Jason Aronson, 1987.
A collection of Gregory Bateson's writings on cybernetics, biology, psychology and epistemology.

Chopra, Deepak, *Quantum Healing: Exploring the Frontiers of Mind/ Body Medicine*, Bantam, 1989.
This book suggests connections between physiology, thought and an embodied network of intelligence.

DeLozier, Judith and Grinder, John, *Turtles All the Way Down*, Grinder, DeLozier and Associates, 1987.

John Grinder's work on physiological states and perceptual positions.

Dilts, Robert, Hallbom, Tim and Smith, Suzi, *Beliefs: Pathways to Health and Well-Being*, Metamorphous Press, 1990.

The connections between beliefs and health and how NLP can influence both for the better.

Grinder, John and Bandler, Richard, *The Structure of Magic 2*, Science and Behaviour Books, 1975.

The first publication of Bandler and Grinder's work on representational systems.

Huxley, Aldous, *The Perennial Philosophy*, Harper & Row, 1944.

A collection of historical writings on the spiritual life.

O'Connor, Joseph and Seymour, John, *Introducing NLP*, Aquarian, 1993.

A comprehensive guide and overview of NLP.

Shree Purohit Swami, trans. Yeats, W. B., *The Ten Principal Upanishads*, Faber, 1937.

One of the principle texts of Eastern mysticism and spirituality.

ABOUT THE AUTHORS

Joseph O'Connor

Joseph O'Connor is an international author, trainer, executive coach and consultant. He is a leading author and trainer in coaching and neuro-linguistic programming (NLP) and systemic thinking. He is the author of 18 books and three audiotapes on coaching, NLP, training, sales communication skills, management and systemic thinking. His books have been translated into 29 languages and have sold half a million copies worldwide.

He is co-founder of the International Coaching Community (ICC), co-founder and director of ROI Coaching, specialist coaching for financial executives, co-founder of the Master Coach Academy Europe, and he is Visiting Professor of Coaching, ISCTE University Business School, Lisbon, Portugal. He spent many years as a professional classical guitarist and has an LRAM from the Royal Academy of Music. He lives in London now, having spent eight years living in Sao Paulo, Brazil.

Contact Joseph at www.lambent.com.

Books by Joseph O'Connor

How Coaching Works with Andrea Lages (AC Black, 2007)

Coaching with NLP with Andrea Lages (Thorsons, 2005)

Free Yourself from Fears (Nicholas Brealey, 2005)

The NLP Workbook (Thorsons, 2001)

NLP and Sports (Thorsons, 2000)
(also available as an ebook)

Extraordinary Solutions for Everyday Problems (Thorsons, 1999)
(also available as an ebook)

Leading with NLP (Thorsons, 1998)

NLP and Health with Ian McDermott (Thorsons, 1997)
(also available as an ebook)

The Art of Systems Thinking with Ian McDermott (Thorsons, 1997)
(also available as an ebook)

First Directions with Ian McDermott (Gower, 1996)

Practical NLP for Managers with Ian McDermott (Gower, 1996)
(also available as an ebook)

Successful Selling with NLP with Robin Prior (Thorsons, 1995)

Training with NLP with John Seymour (Thorsons, 1994)

Introducing Neuro-Linguistic Programming with John Seymour
(Thorsons, 1990)

Not Pulling Strings (Lambent Books, 1987)

Audiobooks

Leading with NLP (Thorsons, 1999)

NLP and Health with Ian McDermott (Thorsons, 1998)

Introducing NLP with Ian McDermott (Thorsons, 1995)

Ian McDermott

Ian McDermott was attracted to NLP because he wanted to know how people who achieved outstanding results did so. He hoped that this know-how could be codified into skill sets. He wanted to then make this available to others and so raise performance in just about any area of human endeavour.

Ian is a UKCP-accredited psychotherapist and also a Diplomate of the International Academy of Behavioral Medicine, Counseling and Psychotherapy. Named one of Britain's Top 10 Coaches and described as 'the Coaches' Coach' (*The Independent*) he has spent the past decade training the next generation of coaches. A thought leader in the field of leadership coaching, and the author of 15 books on NLP, coaching and systems thinking, Ian has a global perspective from working with international companies such as Shell, BP, GSK, FQML and EY. He is also on the Association for Coaching's Global Advisory Panel.

From practical experience he knows what it takes to run a long-term successful business: he founded International Teaching Seminars (ITS) in 1988 which continues to prosper and to pioneer the practical applications of the latest neural research (see below). His work is featured in the Open University's MBA course 'Creativity, Innovation and Change'.

Appointed External Faculty at Henley Business School, he is one of the founding faculty responsible for creating the Henley MSc in Coaching and Behavioural Change. Ian is also an Honorary Fellow of Exeter University Business School, where his focus is on entrepreneurship and innovation. His next book, co-authored with Professor John Bessant, is on how individuals and organizations can become more innovative.

He continues to work with global teams as well as with individual clients.

Contact Ian at www.itsnlp.com.

Books by Ian McDermott

Boost Your Confidence (Piatkus, 2010)
(also available as an ebook)

The Coaching Bible with Wendy Jago (Piatkus, 2005)
(also available as an ebook)

Your Inner Coach with Wendy Jago (Piatkus, 2003)
(also available as an ebook)

Brief NLP Therapy with Wendy Jago (Sage, 2001)
(also available as an ebook)

The NLP Coach with Wendy Jago (Piatkus, 2001)
(also available as an ebook)

First Directions NLP with Joseph O'Connor (Thorsons, 2001)
(also available as an ebook)

Manage Yourself, Manage Your Life with Ian Shircore (Piatkus, 1999)
(also available as an ebook)

NLP and the New Manager with Ian Shircore (Texere, 1998)
(also available as an ebook)

The Art of Systems Thinking with Joseph O'Connor (Thorsons, 1997)
(also available as an ebook)

NLP and Health with Joseph O'Connor (Thorsons, 1996)
(also available as an ebook)

Practical NLP for Managers with Joseph O'Connor (Thorsons, 1996)
(also available as an ebook)

Take Control of Your Life with Joseph O'Connor *et al.* (Time-Life, 1996)

Develop Your Leadership Qualities with Joseph O'Connor *et al.* (Time-Life, 1995)

Audiobooks

Boost Your Confidence (Piatkus, 2010)

Essential Coaching Skills (ITS, 2004)

How to Coach Yourself (ITS, 2004)

Spiritual Dimension of Coaching (ITS, 2004)

The Power to Change (ITS, 2004)

NLP: Health and Well Being with Joseph O'Connor (Thorsons/HarperCollins, 1998)

Professional Development Programme (ITS, 1997)

Tools for Transformation (ITS, 1996)

An Introduction to NLP: Psychological Skills for Understanding and Handling People with Joseph O'Connor (HarperCollins, 1996)

Freedom from the Past (ITS, 1995)

About International Teaching Seminars

Ian McDermott founded International Teaching Seminars (ITS) in 1988 to provide practical skills-based training in effective change technologies for individuals and organizations in both the public and private sector. Systems thinking, NLP and coaching have been the primary vehicles for doing this.

ITS is home to many of the leading figures in the field and is recognized by credible third parties such as Henley Business School as the place to go for training. ITS programmes attract people from all over the world.

ITS is an ISO 9001 certified organization and has international recognition as an accredited coach training provider from the International Coach Federation, the largest body overseeing coaching standards in the world. To learn more about training possibilities and the ITS Career Path, visit www.itsnlp.com or call +44 (0)1268 777125.

INDEX